Practical Guide to Far-Eastern Macrobiotic Medicine

George Ohsawa

Compiled by Herman Aihara

George Ohsawa Macrobiotic Foundation
Chico, California

Practical Guide to Far-Eastern Macrobiotic Medicine was compiled by Herman Aihara in 1976 from George Ohsawa's writings and teachings. It contains the macrobiotic viewpoints at that time. Even though there are many ideas and remedies that may be beneficial, it is important to realize that all things change and current thinking should be consulted.

Also, the information and advice contained in this book are based upon the research and experiences of George Ohsawa. They are not intended as a substitute for consulting with a health care professional. The publisher is not responsible for any adverse effects or consequences resulting from the use of any of the suggestions, preparations, or procedures discussed in this book. All matters pertaining to physical health should be supervised by a health care professional.

This book is made possible through a generous donation from Helen and Michael Fisher.

Cover design by Carl Campbell
Text layout and design by Carl Ferré

First Edition	1976
Current Printing: edited and reformatted	2010 Sep 1

© copyright 1976 by
George Ohsawa Macrobiotic Foundation
    PO Box 3998, Chico, California 95927-3998
    530-566-9765; fax 530-566-9768; *gomf@earthlink.net*
    www.ohsawamacrobiotics.com

Published with the help of East West Center for Macrobiotics
    www.eastwestmacrobiotics.com

ISBN 978-0-918860-21-7

Contents

Foreword

This book, a compilation of several books and writings of George Ohsawa, attempts to give the whole scope of macrobiotic medicine to everyone. The main part is treatment for sickness. However, treatment without understanding principles and having a good attitude is dangerous. Therefore, the theory of macrobiotics and other articles were added. The book, like its predecessor, *The Unique Principle*, is unique not because of its name and contents, but rather in how it was translated, edited, and published.

The first part is a translation taken from Japanese books such as *A New Dietetic Cure, How to Cure Sickness and a Sick Man*, and *Vegetarianism*. The second part is a translation from the French edition of *Practical Guide to Far-Eastern Medicine,* which was done by Ann Harris. Noburo Muramoto was consulted to suit remedies to present-day American needs.

Cornellia Aihara translated *Cooking for the Sick,* which was written by Lima Ohsawa. *Massage and Hand Healing* are based on notes taken by Cynthia McCluskey at Mirimichi Summer Camp, 1972. Photographs of Cornellia demonstrating external treatments were taken by Fred Pulver. *The Manual of Macrobiotics* is a contribution of Nina Bond who took notes at George Ohsawa's lectures in New York at Summer Camp held in 1961.

The third part is a translation from French and Japanese by Fred Pulver, Lou Oles, and Herman Aihara.

The last part is again taken from several articles appearing in past issues of *The Macrobiotic* magazine. The Appendix is taken from a translation of the French edition of Ohsawa's *Practical Guide to Far-Eastern Medicine.*

For beginners, we recommend reading *Macrobiotics: An Invitation to Health and Happiness* before this book. In addition, *The Unique Principle* and *Philosophy of Oriental Medicine* are also of great value for those who want to study further macrobiotic principles. For the sick, we recommend keeping in contact with experienced macrobiotic persons and centers.

We hope this book can be a guide to all macrobiotic people, old and new, for curing sickness and maintaining health and happiness. To realize this book, enormous time and effort was contributed. Special thanks to Tom Goldwasser, Susan Jacobowitz, Maya Edwards, Matthew and Livia Davis, Joe and Mimi Arseguel, and Barbara Grace for their contributions; to Michael Johnston for layout of the book; to Nan Schleiger for art work; to Marvin Mattelson for cover design; and to the staff of the George Ohsawa Macrobiotic Foundation.

Unending thanks to George and Lima Ohsawa.

– Herman Aihara
Editor, 1973

Preface

I am very happy to give you this short, simplified translation of my book, *Cure—Following the New Way of Eating*. It was originally written in Japanese and is now in its 465th edition. I want to share with you the practical application of Macrobiotic healing that I have been teaching for almost 40 years—leaving aside the conceptual aspects covered in my other books and classes.

Herein is the synthesis of my medical philosophy, which is nothing but the biological, physiological, and dialectic interpretation of Far Eastern philosophy—the principles of the Order of the Universe and the Order of Man. For 30 years, I have been writing on both the practical and theoretical sides of this question and have published more than 20 books and thousands of articles. But, at this time, I wish to limit myself to giving easily accessible information.

My medical philosophy, the way of eating and the art of longevity and rejuvenation, is so simple and inexpensive that anyone can follow it any time, anywhere. If you decide to cure yourself before all else, you can forget about the bitter, painful, and costly suffering that results from medical, physical, psychological, and religious therapies.

This system depends on you alone. No reliance on other people or on artificial means—everything depends on how you eat. My system relies more on the sensitization of common sense and morality than on prescribed remedies. It goes to the root rather than treating the symptoms.

The goals of my method are to reach, first, the basis of all disease and, second, the basis of all happiness. So, if you follow the principles of my medicine, you will not only avoid sickness and even un-happiness but also be immune to them in the future. In fact, this new and simplified interpretation of Far Eastern philosophy applied to biology and physiology leads you to eternal happiness, infinite free-dom, absolute integrity, and cosmic love, all through Satvic eating (*Bhagavad-Gita* XVII). Moreover, without this key interpretation, you will never understand these philosophies and their practices—including medicine—and these religions—Christianity, Buddhism, Hinduism, etc.

The great men of today's world are trying to establish peace at home and abroad but, just as in the story of the Tower of Babel, all their efforts, one after the other, fail. The history of human society from the beginning has been a long, a very long, series of failures and reformations—all because men tried to reach peace, happiness, and freedom through force—social, political, economic, or intellec-tual.

A few tried more unorthodox schemes, unprecedented and cruel. Apparently, they forgot that in this relative world what has a begin-ning has an end; and the bigger the back, the bigger the front! They forgot that this temporal and relative world is only a geometric point in the absolute eternal and infinite universe and that it is ruled by the laws of this universe. They could never reach a life of lasting happiness, health, and freedom either for themselves or for others. Instead, they forced other people through the most violent forms of life and death.

Mahatma Gandhi alone, in recent times, denied the value of such systems and relied on nonviolence, fasting, and Ahimsa [biological as well as social pacifism, the embracing of all life, total lack of exclusiveness, infinite gratitude, *on*, which comes from understand-ing the complementary nature of yin and yang—of self to other, the basis of Lao-tse's virtue]. These are our biological, physiological, and dialectical resources. He was a true and brave believer who tried to negate the force of violence even in medicine. Unfortunately, his people's struggle for liberation weighed too heavily on him for him to formulate a modern interpretation of the ancient Oriental wisdom.

Dr. Albert Schweitzer also, as a disciple of one of the most important religions of the East, practiced nonviolence in medicine [See *Book of Cancer*]. But, like Gandhi, Schweitzer did not have the time to study the principle of principles, that of life, the Vedanta, or Chinese philosophy (his medical and biological know-how suffered in proportion to this lack of understanding). There is a Chinese proverb that says: first make a free and peaceful man, then turn to his family, then society; and finally, based on these three, world government. We cannot ignore this sequence. Western socialism, Soviet communism, the various doctrines of anarchy, the utopian theories of Robert Owen, Saint-Simon, and Fourier all attempted to establish freedom and peace, but they did not know how to make free individuals. The lives of their founders were only relatively free; these men did not see that social and group freedom necessarily depends on the freedom of the individual members.

Total ignorance of the Order of the Universe!

On the other hand, all the great and free men of the East (the saints and the prophets) emphasize this Order over and over. Their teachings are forgotten today. So I feel compelled to present a new view of the thousand-years' wisdom and philosophy of China, contemporary in its expression, its aesthetics, its biology, physiology, and dialectics.

Enough theory.

Study and try my way of eating, which is very simple.

Introduction

New Trend in Medicine

Time magazine, April 26, 1947 reports:

For the first time after World War II, medical authorities of the world gathered in New York City. In this conference, Dr. John A. Ryle, a professor of Oxford University, School of Medicine, declared, 'It is time to change microscopic medicine to a macroscopic medicine. The time has come when we must consider man as a member of a family, and a society, when we must relate diseases with living style and livelihood. We are ignorant about the important factors in health and sickness. For example:

1. What are the conditions which produce health in man?
2. Why has stomach ulcer increased in the 20th century?
3. Why did the death rate and the number of tuberculosis victims decrease during wartime even though the food supply was less at that time?
4. Why did laborers die from stomach ulcer or skin cancer at a rate twice as high as did technicians?
5. Why did doctors die from constriction of the heart 12 times more than farmers?

At the same conference Dr. Sir Holden, professor of Baltromey hospital said, 'Doctors must write prescriptions for health but not for sickness. Future doctors must be educators and less treaters. Doctors must work so that a healthy person can stay healthy and not change the sick to the weak.

This report tells me that the new trend in medicine is favorable for my interpretation, which I have been proclaiming for more than 40 years. I will be able to resign from the field of medicine soon. Before I retreat from the medical field, I am writing this book as a practical summary of the Macrobiotic medicine by which thousands of people recovered their health. I intend to write in this book not only to show you how to cure sickness but also to show you how to be happy. Without happiness, health has no value. A way to happiness has been attempted by many for thousands of years. My way is different from all of them. My way is to establish biological and physiological health first and then psychological and spiritual health—happiness.

Most sages of the past taught the way to happiness through psychological and spiritual development or discipline. On this point also, my way is unique. This book is my humble expression of wishes that you will be able to attain health and happiness through the simple dietary and spiritual observations that thousands of people have done.

"I will Give You a Key to the Kingdom of Heaven"
(Matthew 16:19)

This book is a condensation of what I taught for 40 years, through various writings and lectures. What I write here is a secret by which you can cure not only diseases but also unhappiness, such as accidents, injuries, misfortunes, fear, sufferings, insecurity, etc. In other words, I am writing here about a way by which one can live his life freely, peacefully, joyously, and gratefully. How pitiful for someone to have accidents or disasters even though he is healthy! However, a really healthy person never has an accident or a disaster because he has a healthy intuition that foresees the coming disaster and enables him to prevent or escape such occurrences. A healthy person will not suffer even though he meets accidents. I have had many accidents or miseries, including twice the death sentence. Each time I managed to escape miraculously. I guarantee you that you will not meet any accidents or miseries or sufferings from such accidents, if you follow my directions faithfully. However, the prevention or cure of sickness or accidents is not my only wish for writing this, it is also to enable you to establish happiness.

I think the happy life is to live joyfully doing whatever one likes to do during his whole life. In fact, everyone has been living like this. The only trouble is that most of them are not able to continue this way of living because of accidents or suffering from sicknesses. At every minute of our life, we face a decision of choice that is made by our will. We seldom lack the freedom of choice. If we don't have the freedom of choice, we will fight with our whole strength and effort, as seen in man's history. If this is the case, why are most of us not happy? The reason for this is simple—We are not making the right selection in choosing mates, jobs, books, friends, and eating and drinking. We choose something that gives us temporal pleasure but not eternal joy. This temporal pleasure turns to sadness according to the Law of Nature.

I call the selecting or judging ability, which brings us the eternal joy, the Supreme Judgment or Wisdom. Judgment has six stages. The judgment which brings us temporal pleasure is the lowest judgment (see *Macrobiotics: An Invitation to Health and Happiness*). Therefore, in order to live the joyful life by doing only what we like to do, we need to have a higher judgment—if not the Supreme Judgment. Many wise men of the East as well as the West have taught about the Supreme Judgment. Christianity, with millions of followers, has the most famous one—the Key to the Kingdom of Heaven of the Bible. Lao-tse taught the Supreme Judgment as Wu Wei (live according to the Order of the Universe). Confucius taught moderation. Buddha taught the Middle Way. Of course, there are numerous teachings in the West too. However, few of them taught how to choose foods, which, in fact, are our physiological and psychological foundation. Without foods, there is no life. Right foods or diet bring us health, and bad foods or diet bring us sickness and unhappiness. Therefore, judgment that chooses right foods is a basic and fundamental factor of our happiness and health. I call this judgment the "Unique Principle." It will enable you to have the Supreme Judgment in every minute and in every domain of life. The Unique Principle is the modernization of a 5,000-year-old Oriental philosophy or way of thinking. The Unique Principle is the Key to the Kingdom of Heaven taught by Christ. The practical application of the Unique Principle is the macrobiotic diet and medicine about which I am writing here.

Part 1

Theory of Macrobiotic Medicine

How Did I Find Macrobiotics? The Principle of Life

I was born at Sagano, Kyoto, Japan in 1893. My mother could not produce enough milk, and I was a weak baby. I was told by mother that I almost died five times before I reached the first birthday. My family was poor. Father was a principal of an elementary school of a small village before I was born. Then my parents moved to Kyoto where he became a policeman. Mother worked at home to help finance—making strings for kimonos. Mother was an industrious woman. She studied Western science and culture through Yuzuru Niijima who was the founder of the Doshisha University. She died at the age of 30 from tuberculosis, leaving two sons. I was 10 and a younger brother was 6. Two sisters had died earlier due to the wrong diet, which my mother introduced in our family through her study of Western science and culture.

From that time, we lived sad days as poor orphans. I was an apprentice in a Buddhist temple as a disciple. However, I soon started to vomit blood like my mother and sisters had. At 18, I had to give up my school, medicine, eggs, and meat because I was too poor to continue such expensive living. I lived in the lowest living condition. In other words, I lived with brown rice, radish pickle, and salt plum even though I was told by the doctors that my sickness—tuberculosis—required eggs and meats. And my mother gave us milk, eggs, and bread every morning, which was violating natural order.

We were punished for this violation. Such a diet destroyed our family's health. I, however, resented that I could not afford to continue such a diet because I didn't know the fact that such a diet was the cause of mother's and sisters' deaths and my sickness. If I could have afforded to continue that diet, I would have died at that time. I am so grateful that I was poor.

This story may sound strange to you. Life is strange and miraculous. Without miracles, there is no life. I have written many books and articles for over 40 years about the secrets of how I cured my diseases and led a happy life. By this secret, I cured thousands of the sick. My book on this diet sold millions of copies in Japan. This book is an English edition of my Japanese publication—*The New Macrobiotic Medicine.*

Curing all my diseases and re-establishing my health at the age of 20, I realized that food is the source of life. After realization of this important fact, I decided to devote my life to preaching this doctrine. My devotion to this doctrine, however, caused strong antagonisms such as accusations from the public, the medical society and the police. I was tortured by police several times. Publication of my books was stopped several times. My decision to work on Macrobiotic medicine, however, never changed. Starting as a clerk in a trading company, I became a manager and then the president. During this time, I supported my father and my step-mother—giving them one-third of my income. I spent the rest of the income on my life work—the Macrobiotic movement, which included publishing a monthly magazine, over 200 books, the distribution of macrobiotic foods, operating cooking classes, giving lectures, organizing summer schools, camps, and restaurants, etc.

I traveled to France for the first time in 1914. Since then, I have returned a dozen or more times to transplant the unifying principle of Far Eastern science and philosophy—the matrix of all eastern religions and civilizations—and to set up a deep and meaningful understanding between the East and the West. But, to my sadness, I convinced no one. So I had to earn my living teaching and practicing acupuncture and introducing the art of flower arrangement, Buddhism, bonsai, bonkei, the theory behind Judo, etc. I could not go on like that.

At the age of 35, I quit businesses in Japan and went to Europe with 200 yen pocket money only in order to confirm my belief—the secret of life for health and happiness.

In Europe, in order to explain macrobiotics to Westerners, I first studied science. I lived at the lowest standard of living. However, I cured many sick people by Macrobiotic medicine. During my first year in Paris, I published the *Unique Principle*, which is my first publication and explains the principle of the Oriental philosophy. Six years later, I went back to Japan where the political situation was very tense, and Japanese militarism was taking over the government. I intentionally consulted many noble families and intellectuals in order to avoid military pressure. The outbreak of the Sino-Japanese War prohibited my return to Europe.

Since I had studied the principle of Change—Yin-Yang—I often made prophecies in many fields such as personal futures, social problems, world situations, etc. Later I made prophecies that Japan would be defeated and the government leaders shot. This prophecy was realized later. Due to my prophecies concerning the future of Japan and Japanese government, I was arrested several times. My publications were stopped, and my institution was closed by the military government. Finally, I was sentenced to death twice, and it was General McArthur who released me from execution at the last minute. As soon as I was released from the jail, I started activities on Macrobiotic education in Japan hoping to find a few young Japanese who would be able to understand Macrobiotics and the Unique Principle. From these activities, a few Japanese youth followed me and went to Europe, North America, India, and South America—these included Michio Kushi, Aveline Kushi, Clim Yoshimi, Tomio Kikuchi, Abe Nakamura, Herman Aihara, Cornellia Aihara, etc.

In 1953, at age 60, I left Japan for India—to teach Macrobiotics to the world.

Now, I am returning to France, 20 years after leaving, and after two years in India and eight months in Equatorial Africa. And now, I, the first practitioner-importer of acupuncture into Europe, am overwhelmed at the sight of hundreds of acupuncturists "made in France"! Books on Buddhism and Japanese architecture, masters of flower arrangement, thousands of Judo-kas, bonkei in the 5 and 10's! This is why I speak so urgently to you of the Unifying Principle of Yin and Yang. Without this basic understanding, you will be lost in any Far Eastern scientific and philosophic studies. Even though I was very sick in my youth, I lived a most exciting life, enjoying my life, curing thousands of the sick, and changing unhappy ones into happy ones. This book is a practical guide for living for whoever wishes to live such an exciting and wonderful life. Such persons must understand the following poem.

> For one who has no sadness, there is no joy.
> For one who has joy, sadness follows.
> Overcoming sadness and suffering.
> Come to the land
> Where there is eternal joy.

What is Your Aim in Life?

Please write down your answer to the above question before reading my answer which follows.

One day, a 50-year-old lady came to see me. Her husband, an ex-president of a big hospital, was dying with heart disease. She lost all her fortune and the hospital by air bombing during World War II. Now she was losing her husband. "I am a Christian. I lived my life for other's sake as taught in the Bible. I helped many people. Why should I suffer from such miseries when I was doing good?" she asked me.

I answered her, "You had a wrong idea about your aim in life. You said that you lived for others. This is a wrong idea. Nobody likes to do something for others really. Everyone wants to do for himself. In other words, so-called altruists are doing what they want to do. Everyone likes to eat delicious foods, to take good sleep, to live in a luxurious home with leisure time. There are no real altruists. One who thinks he works for others is a liar. You are a liar. You have lived a lie for 40 years. Therefore, you are unhappy now. You must live doing what you like to do most."

Another lady came to consult me. She graduated from a university and married an ideal man whom she loved. They lived together 25 years without much difficulties. She is 55 years old now, and she found her life was not interesting. Her husband goes to the company routinely every morning, where he has an important job, and comes back home at night. His only pleasure is to drink sake and sleep. She feels her life is like a machine or the life of a slave. What a sad life when someone finds himself living as a slave after 25 years of ideal life.

A businessman who established a big trading company after many years of hard work came to see me. At age 65, he lost his business and his only son by the war. His wife had cancer. At age 65 he had to cook and care for his wife. What a sadness.

I met many unhappy people but few happy ones. Where is a happy life? Those people had a wrong aim in their life. Therefore, they ended up their life unhappy. According to my 35 years of teaching toward health and happiness, I concluded that without health there is no happiness. All unhappiness—poverty, misery, failure with business, family trouble, and accidents—are the result of unhealthiness. Without health, any success in life will not last long. Without knowing how to be healthy, happiness is illusion. There are some healthy persons who are not happy. They are, however, not really healthy. Their health was given by their parents but not made by themselves. Health must be made by yourself. Such health only is yours. One who makes himself healthy knows the law of change. Therefore, he can overcome the difficulties. He can change sickness to health, sadness to joy, and enemy to friend. He is a free man. This is my aim in life—to be a free man. To be a man, you must discipline yourself to be healthy. If you cannot free yourself from sickness, you cannot be a free man. You will end up a slave—a slave to wages, a slave to status, a slave to medicine, and a slave to fame.

Now I have to define the term of health as I know it—which is quite different from so-called health.

What is Health?

I define health with six conditions. These conditions consist of three physiological conditions and three psychological ones—as explained in *Macrobiotics: An Invitation to Health and Happiness*. They are as follows:

1. Never tired. Always ready to do something.   10 points
2. Good appetite. Enjoy and be satisfied with the simplest meal at any time.   10 points
3. Good sleep. Sleep within three minutes after going to bed. Never waking up to go to the bathroom. Never having nightmares. Not talking while sleeping. Waking up at a set time and finish washing your face within three minutes. Waking up in the same position as when you started sleeping. Four hours of sleeping is enough.   10 points
4. Good memory.   20 points
5. Joyous, never angry. Making people happy and joyful.   20 points
6. Neatness in everything, everywhere and in every way.   <u>30 points</u>

Total   100 points

Minus conditions: Shoulder stiffness, catching cold, wearing eye glasses before you are 50 years old. Irregular menstruation. One who does not menstruate every 28 days. Grey hair before you are 50 years old.   - 10 points

Translator's Note: Ohsawa added a 7th condition to the above six when he was in New York City in 1962, which appeared in his letter to the Japanese Macrobiotics in Tokyo. He says in his letter as follows:

> I had coined six conditions of health about 30 years ago. Since then, no one revised it. Now I am adding a 7th condition to it. With this condition, I have to give a new way of counting. The first three conditions count 5 points each. The last three conditions count 10 points each. The rest—55 points—goes to the 7th condition because it is more important than the other six conditions combined. The 7th condition of health is a result of my 40 years of macrobiotic teaching. This finding was triggered by Mr. G., who gave me a chance to learn the most important condition of health. He is one of my oldest and loyalest disciples. He attended my lectures for more than 20 years. Recently, I was shocked by his attitude in which he took for granted his child's lie as a matter of fact. He has no responsibility about honesty or justice. He has no sense of integrity. He seemed to think lying is not bad at all. After this incident, I looked at him more carefully. As a result, I noticed that he is very suspicious, rigid, mean, and holds hidden anger. In short, he is not healthy at all. Why could he not establish health after observing the macrobiotic diet for more than 20 years? After thinking several months, I reached the conclusion that he lacked the 7th condition of health—absolute honesty.

The 7th condition of health is extremely important. It is more important than the other six conditions combined. The six conditions are included in the 7th condition. One who observes the 7th condition is more healthy than one who has attained all the other conditions. On the other hand, one who has not attained the 7th condition cannot be healthy however much he may have mastered the others. Then what is the 7th condition of health?

The 7th condition of health is righteousness or integrity. According to *Encyclopedia Americana*, "Integrity is like happiness, something never realized." According to Eastern philosophy, Integrity is the foundation of the Universe and life. It is the principle of life, Tao, the Order. It is the spirit, God, Atman. If Integrity is explained in practical terms, it will be the following state of mind.

A. Be grateful for everything, even for difficulties, poverty, unhappiness, and sickness.

B. Be neither fearful nor angry any time about anything.

C. Have faith in the Order of the Universe. Do not give up. Do not become frustrated.

D. Do not forget what you receive in favors and kindness or help from others. And always try to show appreciation.

E. Never lie in order to protect yourself.

F. Be exact.

G. Like everyone. Live with the motto, "I never met a man I didn't like."

H. Never be suspicious of others.

I. Never pretend to be altruistic.

J. Always find great joy in unimportant things.

K. Give to others what is most important to you.

L. Understand that life is a miracle, and everyone has the ability to create that miracle. That I am living is a miracle. This realization is justice. One who has reached this realization can realize anything. This is the spiritual power. Without this spiritual power, one cannot cure disease. Without this spiritual power, one cannot be happy.

Macrobiotic medicine is a technique to lead you to this spiritual power, which, in fact, you already have. If you have no will to realize this miracle, this book is of no use. If you have no idea what you want to do with your health, curing sickness is wasting time. To realize this spiritual power of Justice (Integrity) in our life is curing.

Judgment—The Ultimate Cause of Sickness

The cause of all unhappiness and disease exists in our lower judgment or eclipsed judgment. However hard we try to cure sickness, it is in vain unless we improve our judgment. This is my conclusion after 40 years of curing many sick people.

Improving our judgment is very difficult. Arnold Toynbee said in his famous book, *The Study of History*, that in man's history 20 civilizations have already fallen, and five more are diminishing. This is the proof that all civilizations were built by poor judgment. All religions, such as Christianity, Hinduism, Islam, Buddhism, Confucianism, Taoism, and Shintoism are aiming at improving one's Judgment so that one can come to know infinite freedom, eternal happiness, and absolute justice (integrity).

Western democracy has a similar purpose to that of Eastern religion. The difference between the two is in the fact that the former aims at the greatest happiness of the majority while the latter aims at eternal happiness for everyone. Therefore, they are entirely different teachings, or opposite ways of life. Freedom in the democratic society is achieved by slavery or exploitation. In other words, someone's freedom is another one's unfreedom. Its happiness is based on money, matter, or comfort. Therefore, happiness is limiting and ephemeral. Its justice is based on the law that always creates outlaws or protesters because it protects only the majority but not the right. The logic used in the democratic society is dualistic, formal logic, but it is not applicable to the Infinite or the World of Spirit. The medicine in the democratic world is egoistic. It serves humans but not bacteria virus. They think they can kill any living thing in order to save the human. Therefore, the more that Western democracy progresses the more man becomes unfree, sick, unjust, explosive and violent. Everyday's news proves this. The Eastern world adopted Western democracy and is following in the footsteps of the tragedy of the Western world. Sir James Brice, the author of *Modern Democracies*, said, "The real democracy of man will be completed when man knows himself." These words are the same as those of Alexis Carrel in *Man, The Unknown*. Thomas Edison, the famous inventor, cried in his later years saying that we acquired so much knowledge, invented machines to make life comfortable, and conquered nature, but our health, happiness, freedom, and peace had not improved at all. George Eastman, the founder of Kodak Company, committed suicide saying that life is not interesting. John D. Rockefeller Sr., who donated $600 million in his lifetime died from stomach ulcer at the age of 98, even though he offered half his fortune to such a person, he searched in vain for someone who might be able to cure his sickness. Were these rich and successful people happy? Is it impossible to establish happiness in this world?

In contrast to the West, the East approaches happiness, freedom, and justice in an entirely different way. It seems to me that even though they didn't invent many comfortable machines nor exploit the new world, they enjoyed a happier and more peaceful life, as Lin Yutang has said. However, I am not a man who is against science, industry, nor democracy. I am merely offering the Eastern way of thinking and its practical application to living. Eastern people approached happiness by the way of improving their thinking or judgment. I will explain what I mean by judgment.

All conflict comes from misunderstanding between two or more people. All misunderstanding comes from the fact that one does not explain his thinking clearly enough or adequately enough so that others are able to understand what he is saying. Another cause of misunderstanding is in the fact that we lack proper words or concepts to communicate our thinking or feeling to others exactly as we think. For example, if I say this food is sweet, I am thinking others will taste the same sweetness more or less that I taste. Often we find that this is not always true. Our tasting perception is very individualistic. In the same way, what I like may be another's dislike. This will lead to sentimental misunderstanding and then conflict. This misunderstanding is highly critical in the case of religion or morals. Arab and Jewish people have misunderstood each other for thousands of years. They are still fighting each other.

Because nobody has the same knowledge, same taste, feeling, or belief, how can we avoid the conflict that is the result of misunderstanding or miscommunication. For this, we should have higher thinking or judgment. Tensin Okakura, the author of *The Book of Tea*, said, "If you become a little higher in judgment, then you will have no difficulties at all in the future." If you can't judge, you can't live. Even your heart is judging, expanding, and contracting. (This antagonistic movement is very important.) All our functions are judgment. There is nothing but judgment in this world. The philosophy of the East is judgment or thinking (Prajna). Someone told me that thinking is not respected in this country. This shocked me very much because I came to this country to teach you how to think— how to judge in order to be happy and free.

According to the Oriental philosophy, there are two categories of man. The first is he who can judge and think. The other can't think but imitates. Generally speaking, everyone can think but most are accustomed to not thinking. Many borrow the judgment of others. I studied biology 39 years ago in the Pasteur Institute in Paris, especially the anatomy of animals. I found many very interesting

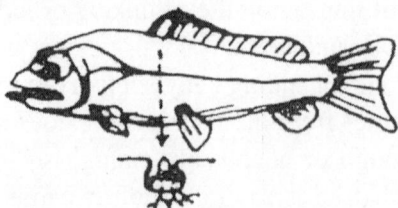

things. For example: fish have a trace of a central sensory system; however, they don't have a big brain. Therefore, they can sense but not think. Dogs and cats have a small brain so that they have a little sentimentality and intellectuality but cannot think as man does. Even in the monkey, the brain is very small. I understood why he can't think. But it is very strange with man. All men have a big brain and yet they can't think—except for a few. [Ohsawa means to think creatively and originally and not merely express knowledge that is the result of others' thinking. Especially his thinking means to think about the Ultimate, God, Totality or Absolute. He thinks that a free, happy man is one who thinks originally. The followers are always imitators, and the imitator is not a creator. He cannot be a happy man. Ohsawa emphasizes the importance of one's own original thinking and not the knowledge that is acquired by school teaching or book reading.]

According to my opinion, judgment has seven stages of expression, which are the result of biological development.

1. The first stage of judgment is the most simple, blind, mechanical judgment such as physical reaction to heat, cold, or pain. This comes a few hours after birth.

2. The second stage of judgment is sensory judgment. A few days after birth the baby develops sensory perception such as light, dark, hunger, and suffering, etc. As the baby grows, this judgment develops further in detailed grades—the judgment of color, shape, temperature, taste, smell, and sound appears. These are sensorial judgments that can be divided into Yin and Yang.

3. The third stage of judgment is sentimental judgment. As the sensorial judgment grows for two to three months, the baby starts to show like-dislike, love-hate, fear-friendliness, etc.

4. The fourth stage of judgment is intellectual judgment. Around 5 years old, children start to show conceptual judgment. This leads to knowledge, abstraction, and synthesis of concepts.

5. The fifth stage of judgment is social judgment. In this stage, judgment reaches beyond oneself—from ego to family, friends, school, etc. This includes two types of judgment. One is moral, and the other is economic. The economic judgment is more powerful than the moral judgment.

6. The sixth judgment is ideological judgment such as religion, socialism, capitalism, and communism. Man is born good antagonizes with man is born bad. Such a basic antagonistic concept is ideological judgment. Optimist and pessimist. One who accepts life and one who negates life. Independent man versus dependent, slavelike man, thinkers versus nonthinkers.

7. The seventh judgment is Supreme Judgment in which one finally opens his eyes for the Order of the Universe; it is the principle that embraces all phenomena and matters.

This is my rough sketch of the stages of judgment. These stages are the *expression* of our judgment and not the judgment itself which existed before birth and has not been changed by physical development. The relationship between judgment and its expression is the same relationship as between memory and our memories. Our memories are stored in our brain cells but the memory is not in our brain. The memory existed before our birth.

Judgment or the 7th level of judgment is the synonym for Universal Consciousness, God, Atman, Taikyoku, Memory, Love, Grace, Infinity, Freedom, Happiness, Health, Justice, etc. [Please see *Unique Principle*, by George Ohsawa.]

Since ancient times, many sages called for the Supreme Judgment saying "Know Yourself," "Know the Truth," "Be Yourself," "Self Realization," "Satori," "Nirvana," "Nenbutsu," and "Nam Myo Ho Ren Ge Kyo," etc. But people didn't understand these words and were surprised when they were told "Be Yourself."

"Am I not Myself?"

"Who am I?" Or,

"Who was I?"

This is a nonsense story like that of Dr. S., who was my patient, to cure his weak memory. One day he was looking for his hat all over the room because he had forgotten the fact that he was wearing the hat on his head.

There are so many federalists and peace-makers who are against war. They are mostly sentimental because they dislike war. They are against war because they lost their son, husband or fortunes, etc. This is a sentimental judgment and, in other words, they are egoists. This low judgment is the cause of war. Krishna of India didn't deny the war (see *Bhagavad-Gita*). The reason wars never disappear from our society is the fact that there are always sentimental, egoistic peace-makers. Also, another reason for the existence of war is the low judgment of politicians. Most politicians are at the second stage of judgment. Their judgment is based on power of money, law, majority, etc. What an irrational judgment to think that peace can be brought by power, bombs, armies, and violence! They are living with lower judgment than gangs who showed the social judgment or even religious judgment following the code of no double talk. There is no end of war until politicians reach the Supreme Judgment.

All judgment except the 7th level is antagonistic, composed of two forces called Yin and Yang by ancient Chinese philosophers. Because Macrobiotic medicine is one level of judgment applied to sickness, I have to explain Yin and Yang before we go further into the details of Macrobiotic medicine.

Yin and Yang
Method of Classification

Five thousand years ago, the Unique Principle of Yin and Yang was a physical dialectic, as it is today. The sky, a boundless expansion of infinite space, was the supreme symbol of Yin, a centrifugal force. The earth—heavy, compact, condensed—was its opposite, Yang, a centripetal force.

The metaphysical application of Yin and Yang reverses the physical. The sky, or heaven, the divine, generates all physical phenomena. Generation (i.e., creation, activity, movement) is the property of Yang; therefore, the sky is Yang. Because the Order of the Universe is in alternation, and the Yang sky produced the earth, it must follow that the earth is Yin.

This metaphysical reversal of Yin and Yang terminology exists throughout much of Chinese literature. Early commentators erroneously affixed metaphysical labels to material phenomena and succeeding chroniclers compounded the confusion.

Even the famous *Nei-Ching, the Yellow Emperor's Classic of Internal Medicine*, classifies the hollow, passive, and receptive Yang, while the dense, compact, and active organs (liver, kidneys, heart) are termed Yin. Such terminology, of course, contradicts the fundamental meanings of Yin and Yang in the physical world.

Lao-Tse, poet of the Unique Principle, in Chapter 42 of the *Tao te Ching* correctly defines Yin and Yang as "shade" and "sun" respectively. Confucius, who had his difficulties with Lao-Tse's dialectics, if we are to believe some historians, nevertheless employed the *Tao te Ching* definition of Yin and Yang in his compilation of the *I Ching*. Modern macrobiotics adheres to his definition.

In India, Radjasic is manly, cruel—Yang. Tamasic is quiet, passive—Yin.

Every conceivable phenomenon, including all the varied phases of human activity (bathing, sleeping, exercise, study, sexual relations) may be classified as Yin or Yang, then coordinated in accordance with its respective proportion of Yin and Yang constituents.

All phenomena in the universe are occasioned by two fundamental forces: Yin, which is centrifugal, and Yang, which is centripetal.

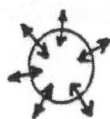

Centrifugal Yin accounts for silence, cold (slackening of the molecular components' activity), dilation, expansion, lightness (i.e., lack of weight)—observe Yin's tendency to rise—tall (vertical) thin forms and darkness.

Centripetal Yang is responsible for manifestations of sound, solid (constriction, density, heaviness)—note Yang's downward direction—flattened, low horizontal forms, heat (activity of the molecular components), and light.

In general, the female Yin (the shade of "the north side of the hill") represents a constellation of the qualities of dark, negative, cold, weak, passive, repose, while the male Yang (the sun of "the south side of the hill") denotes light, positive, heat, strength, active, movement.

However, nothing is wholly Yin or wholly Yang. Everything partakes of both qualities, in proportion. And the proportion is relative. In the scale of Yin and Yang, an object possessing a preponderance of Yang characteristics (e.g., a rock) is deemed Yang. But in relation to a diamond, the most Yang of stones, the rock recedes in Yang value.

Classification of Yin and Yang components is effected (established) by applying the following seven criteria (tests):

1. Physical (color, shape or form, density or weight, temperature, etc.)
2. Chemical (K/Na composition, percentage of water, taste—whether bitter, salty, sour, sweet or pungent, and their chemical, physiological, and biological effect, constrictive or dilative)
3. Biochemical (tropism, autonutrition, heteronutrition, organic, inorganic, morphological, and psychological effects)
4. Bioecological (the influence of such geographical factors as the earth's composition, altitude, climate, configuration, etc.)
5. Historical (the country of origin and adaptability in time and space with reference to geological, geographical, biological, and embryological prospects)
6. Ideological (economic, biological, physiological, medical, sociological, and moral values)
7. The Unique Principle (exercise of humanistic, all-embracing Supreme Judgment)

A. Yin and Yang in Color

We interpret the world through our sensory perceptions—seeing, hearing, tasting, smelling, and touching. Within these, the most important perception is visual perception. In visual perception, we distinguish seven colors that manifest the Order of Nature. I call this Order of Nature Yin and Yang order. You will find this order in every phenomena, and this application in life is very useful and simple. Exercise this classification in many fields before you apply it to medicine, which I am going to write about later in this book.

First of all, you must distinguish yin and yang in color. What color is most yang? What color is most yin?

We define red as yang because it gives us warmth and purple as yin because it gives us a cold feeling. Five colors go between these two yin and yang.

Yang---Yin
Red Orange Brown Yellow Green Blue Violet Purple
7,000 Å (wave length)   4,000 Å (wave length)

We are living between red (yang) and green (yin). Blood is red and vegetables are green. We eat green and it changes to red. We are a transformation of vegetables. Even carnivores depend on the plant world because they eat vegetable eaters. In other words, we live on hemoglobin (▲) which is a product of chlorophyll (▼). Animals are more yang when compared with plants because they have red blood which is yang. However, this yang blood is dependent on the yin plant world. This is the Law of Nature. Yang depends on yin and vice versa.

The disease in which white blood cells increase abnormally and red blood cells decrease is called leukemia or blood cancer. This is a yin disease.

At the end of the second World War, the American Air Force dropped an atomic bomb on Nagasaki where there were two hospitals. One was a Catholic Church Hospital and the other one was Nagasaki University Hospital. The bomb was dropped between these two hospitals. Both were destroyed—3,000 were killed in the University Hospital and 8,000 died on the streets. But no one in Church Hospital was killed nor suffered from leukemia, which is normally caused by the radiation of an atomic bomb. This miracle was caused by my disciple who was a director and doctor of this hospital and kept patients on the Macrobiotic diet. However, the news media did not publicize this fact correctly.

All products of hemoglobin such as meat, eggs, cheese, sausage, etc. are too yang so don't eat too much of these. Biologically speaking, animal foods are not good for our system. On the contrary, if you eat too much purple colored food, you will be yinnized. What food is most purple in color? They are eggplant, tomato, fig, bud of potato, etc. If you have only very yin foods and you don't want to suffer from yin disease, you can yangize them with fire, salt and pressure. We distinguish ourselves from other animals by our use of the invention of fire and salt. No other animals use fire and salt except by natural composition in their food. Human civilization is dependent on the invention of firemaking and on the production of salt.

If you are a vegetarian in this society, you will become so yin that you will be devoured by meat-eaters. You will be happy by yourself, but you will be attacked by meat-eaters. Most vegetarians are idealists and are solitary and retiring.

Infrared rays lie just beyond the red (yang) end of the spectrum and their wave lengths are longer than those of visible light; therefore, they are very yang. Conversely, ultraviolet rays lie beyond the opposite (yin) end of the spectrum, with short wave lengths, and are very yin.

B. Yin and Yang in Water

Is water yin or yang? Is rain yin or yang? When it rains, rheumatics have pain. This is sad and not joyful. So water is yin (cause of yin). Less water is yang. Dry vegetables are more yang than fresh vegetables. Dehydration is yangizing. If you cook vegetables with salt, they expel water and become more yang.

Body metabolic reactions need water. If dehydrated too much, our metabolism slows down and causes a lack of energy. In other words, we need the proper amount of water, which is controlled by the kidneys. Therefore, when our kidneys malfunction, we will be tired. This is an example of yin (water) making yang (energy).

C. Yin and Yang in Chemicals

Na (sodium) is yang and K (potassium) is yin. The body is always balancing these two antagonistic elements. According to my classification of elements, the most yang elements are H (hydrogen), C (carbon), Li (lithium), As (arsenic), and Na. Their wave lengths on the spectroscopic table are longer than 6,000 l (Lambda). The most yin elements are O (oxygen), K (potassium), P (phosphorus), N (nitrogen), Si (silicon), Fe (iron), S (sulfur), Ca (calcium), and B (boron). Their wave lengths are shorter than 4,300 l (Lambda). In between the above-mentioned elements, there are many elements that have different physical and chemical characteristics. They are He (helium), Ne (neon), Mg (magnesium), Cl (chlorine), Cr (chromium), Ni (nickel), Zn (zinc), Pd (palladium), Ag (silver), Hg (mercury), Pt (platinum), and Ge (germanium), etc.

(Please read *Unique Principle* for the further information.)

D. Yin and Yang in Tropism

A plant that grows straight up is yin, and that which grows downward is yang. For example, the upper part of a radish is yin when it is compared with the root. The root is more yang than the upper part.

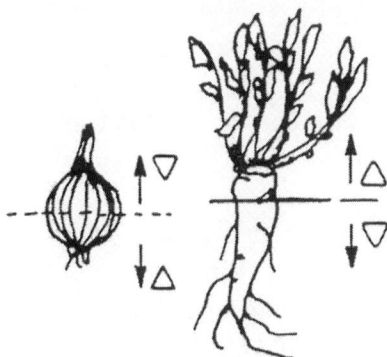

Since any living thing contains more yin elements in the upper parts and more yang elements in the lower parts, we cut onions vertically so that we get both yin and yang elements in our cooking. If we cut horizontally, one piece contains more yang or more yin. And one person may eat more yang onion than another, and one person may eat more yin onion than another. Root vegetables are basically more yang than green vegetables. (See the Appendix for foods listed by yin and yang.)

Growing horizontally under the ground is yin, such as potato. Growing horizontally above the ground is yang, such as dandelion.

A mushroom is very yin—95 percent of it is water. Chinese cooking uses so much meat that lots of mushrooms are used in order to balance with yang meat. Avocados are one of the most yin fruits, so there are more yin sicknesses in countries where avocados grow. Bamboo and sugar cane grow straight up and very fast. They are very yin plants.

E. Yin and Yang in Form (illustration next page)

A, B, C, and D are vertical forms and are governed by yin centrifugal force.

E, F, G, and H are horizontal forms and are dominated by yang centripetal force.

Each vertical form has the same geometric surface as its horizontal opposite but they are antagonistic. The antagonism between forms C and G and forms D and H is marked.

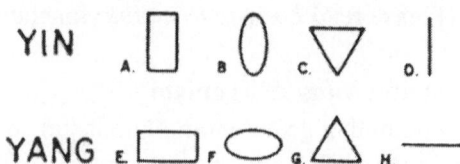

YIN   A. □   B. ◯   C. ▽   D. |

YANG   E. ▭   F. ◯   G. △   H. —

F. Yin and Yang in Weight

Yang centripetal force governs that which is heavy. Yin centrifugal force dominates that which is light.

G. The Summary of Yin and Yang

Yang	Yin
Centripetal force	Centrifugal force
Hot	Cold
Moving	Resting, not moving
Contraction, small	Expansion, large
Downward movement	Upward movement
Short	Long
Dry	Wet
K/Na less than 7:1	K/Na more than 7:1
Animal	Plant
Time	Space
Nucleus, mitocondrium	Protoplasm
Man	Woman

H. Important Notes for Beginners

1. Yin and yang are relative and not absolute. In other words, there is no absolute yin or yang. They are all relative to others. For example, California is west of New York, but east of Tokyo.

2. Yin and yang are changing all the time. The earth is moving with tremendous speed. Our position, environment, season,

and weather are changing at a great speed. Therefore, nothing remains at the same yin and yang balance. For example, radish is watery when it is fresh; it is yin. However, when it is older, it is more yang. If it is dried by the sun, it is more yang. The yin or yang balance changes by the way of cooking, storing, gardening, and cutting.

3. The ratio of K/Na is not an absolute one. It is a mere measuring of factors. Because there are many minerals in our body, you should not judge yin or yang by only this ratio.

4. There are many things that look yang but in reality are yin. For example, when a business is growing, its activities are yang but its expansion indicates yin. If it expands beyond the yang binding power, it falls apart. This is the same in the case of nations. This is the case of "In the extreme, yin produces yang, and yang produces yin." Therefore, we must know whether the particular yin or yang is in its old or young age. If it is in its old age, it may change to the opposite.

   A shape in which the centrifugal force and the centripetal force are balancing is a circle. This is true of any size circle. In other words, yin and yang balance exists from the smallest circle to the largest circle. If the centrifugal force becomes larger than the centripetal force, the circle will expand and then explode. The opposite case will produce contraction. Therefore, we must be careful to balance yin and yang all the time, even though we are balancing perfectly right now. Therefore, when we go to a warmer climate, we eat more yin foods. In a colder climate, we eat more yang foods. It is natural that a yang man wants a yin woman. However, a yin man doesn't want a yin woman, and stays single. Similarly, a yang woman often divorces a yang man because yang repels yang.

5. A yin person becomes yin from eating yin foods or because his mother ate yin foods in her pregnancy. The biological cause of the yang person is the opposite of this example.

6. One who is a balance of small yin and small yang is a yes-

man or square-type person whose character is social and
who keeps a family happy but who is not a great man. He
enjoys being small. One who is a balance of big yin and big
yang will become a great man. He can tolerate difficulties,
embrace that which is disagreeable, and establish a big job.
Each person holds a different grade, or degree, of yin and
yang.

7. Animals or plants that grow bigger in a colder climate are
more yang, and those that grow smaller are more yin. Men,
bears, horses, and crows grow larger in a colder climate;
therefore, they are yang animals. Elephants and monkeys
grow bigger in warmer climates; therefore, they are yin
animals. Giraffes, gorillas, and chimpanzees can live only
in a hot climate. They are very yin animals. White bears live
only in a cold climate because they are very yang. Pine trees
are yang for the same reason.

Classification of Vegetable Foods
in the Northern Hemisphere

	Yang	Yin
Season of growth	▲ Cold (Sep-Feb)	▼ Hot (Mar-Aug)
Speed of growth	Slow	Fast
Direction of growth	Downward, underground	Upward, above ground
Direction of growth at ground level	Horizontal	Vertical
Direction of growth underground	Vertical	Horizontal
Height	Low	High
Water required for growth	Little	Much
Time required to cook	Long	Short
Effect of heat	Harden	Soften

Color	Red, orange, brown, yellow, black	Green, blue, indigo, purple, white
Larger	In the North	In the South

Classification of Animal Foods
in the Northern Hemisphere

	Yang	Yin
Growth	Slow	Fast
Place of growth	Cold	Hot
Action	Fast	Slow
Manner	Active, positive	Passive, negative
Food	Carnivorous fruitarian	Vegetarian,
Water consumption	Little	Much
Face	Square	Long or triangular
Height	Short	Tall
Pulse and respiration	Fast	Slow
Muscle	Hard	Soft
Blood	Concentrated	Less concentrated because of fluid intake
Body temperature	High	Low
Oxygen consumption	Much	Little
Hibernate	Doesn't	Does
Grow larger	North	South

Yin and Yang—The Unique Principle
Translated into 12 Theorems

The seven principles of the Order of the Universe are supplemented by twelve theorems of the Unique Principle. These theorems define the functioning world of relativity:

1. Yin and yang are two poles that come into operation when infinite centrifugality arrives at the geometric point of bifurcation.
2. Yin and yang result continuously from infinite centrifugality.
3. Yin is centrifugal, yang is centripetal. Yin and yang produce energy.
4. Yin attracts yang. Yang attracts yin.
5. Yin and yang combined in varied proportions produce all phenomena.
6. All phenomena are ephemeral, constantly changing their constitutions of yin and yang components.
7. Nothing is exclusively yin or solely yang. Everything is bipolar.
8. There is nothing neutral. Yin or yang is always in changing balance.
9. The force of attraction is proportional to the difference between yin and yang components.
10. Yin repels yin, yang repels yang. Repulsion is inversely proportionate to the difference between yin and yang forces.
11. In the extreme, yin produces yang, and yang produces yin.
12. All phenomena are yang at the center and yin on the surface.

Yin-Yang Physiognomy
Method of Classification

Judgment depends on the quality of the individual cells that compose the body. If these cells are poor quality, then memory and sense reception are clouded and man begins to lose his will to live. When each day the food taken to replace these cells is of poor quality, then each cell grows steadily weaker and weaker. At a certain point, the process must end tragically.

By looking at former President Kennedy's photograph, it is clear that he was very ill. People who understand Macrobiotics knew that he would die tragically. The whole condition of a man—his past, his present, and his future—is written on his face. Former President Johnson's condition was worse. In three years from now, we will see many worse things happen, not only in the United States but all over the world.

From this, we learn the importance of good health. Our condition depends on correct eating and drinking. We do not have to go through misfortune ourselves, for we can learn from others and can take action, directing ourselves to create good health and judgment.

Seeing people is very important. If you know a man's condition, you know a great deal about him. For in his condition is written his past, his present, and his future. To understand this, you must first understand the signs, be able to read them quickly and accurately.

All seeing is related to Yin and Yang, for nothing exists outside of yin and yang. You know the basic qualities of yin—centrifugal, expansion, dark, fragile, delicate, blue, indigo, shy, soft, retiring, cold, liquid, passive, female, contemplative; and of yang—centripetal, contracting, active, forceful, red-yellow, emphatic, material, durable, hot, solid, close to the center of the earth.

Look at the whole of a person. If tall, then more yin. If short, then more yang. If movements are rapid and angular, more yang; if slow and curving, more yin.

Head

The head, the highest body point, is yin. The feet, closer to the earth's center, yang. The brain uses more blood than any other organ. Yin attracts yang.

The spiral or "cowlick" on top of the head is the beginning of life. The body develops from that beginning. Everyone has his spiral; some have two or three.

The front of the head is more yin than the center, the back more yang. If the hair spiral occurs in the center, at the crown of the head, yin and yang were in balance at birth. If the spiral starts towards the front of the head, the person is yin; if towards the back, the person is yang.

The right side of the head is yang, the left yin. The most yang part of the head is located in the back on the right side; the most yin part is in the front on the left side.

What is the shape of the head—round, square, oval, triangular?

The head should be one-seventh the size of the body. If it is smaller than that, the person is yin. The mother's rich yin diet during pregnancy accounts for the diminution. If the head is large, the mother ate a simple, yang diet.

Hair is yin. Baldness and falling hair is caused by excessive yin intake (fruits, sugars, liquids, foods rich in potassium or phosphorus). The scalp is a tight meshwork of yang cells whose function is the nourishment and growth of hair. When these cells are distended by a yin diet, the root of the hair is cast afloat; it literally drowns. Yin repels yin.

Baldness usually begins at the most yin part of the head, in the front. However, if the yin intake includes a quantity of alcohol and drugs, baldness will begin in the back. A bald spot in the center denotes only moderate yinization.

A bulging forehead, or back of the head, is a sign of yin; if either or both are flat, a sign of yang. If the back of the head is flat and the shoulders hunched, the consumption of too much animal protein is indicated. A hunchback is an example.

Face

The face reveals the basic structure. A healthy complexion tends towards the pale side, not flushed or red. Yin factors (sugar, wine, animal protein) will expand the cells, flood the capillaries, and bring blood to the surface of the skin. The cells should be contracted.

If the mother ate a diet in yin/yang balance during pregnancy the facial proportions will be aesthetically pleasing. If there was imbalance, the physiology, character, and temperament of the child will be uneven and confused; his direction will be uncertain, his aims mixed, his goals undefined.

The face should be divisible horizontally into three areas of equal dimensions:

1. From the crown of the head to the top of the eyes;

2. From the top of the eyes to the juncture of the nose and upper lip;

3. From the juncture of the nose and upper lip to the bottom of the chin.

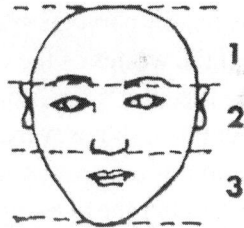

The first area, from the crown of the head to the top of the eyes, contains the hair spiral, where life began *in utero*. This part of the face exhibits the most notable influences of the mother's diet during the first three months of pregnancy. A wide, expanded, or bulging forehead indicates that the maternal nutrition for that three-month period consisted of predominantly yin food. It might be assumed that the date of conception was early summer when yin foods abound. Conversely, a narrow, contracted forehead points to a date of conception in winter when, yin foods being scarce, the mother's main alimentation was yang. But this supposition may prove invalid in a modern metropolis where foods are imported and consumed out of season.

The second area, from the top of the eyes to the juncture of the nose and upper lip, discloses the nature and quality of maternal nutrition during the fourth, fifth, and sixth months of pregnancy.

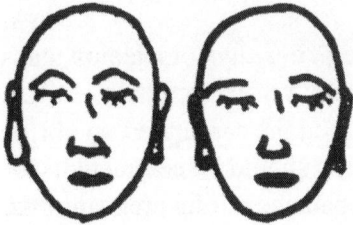

If the eyebrows lie close to the eyes, the mother ate very yang food in the fourth month. When they grow close together above the bridge of the nose then rise in a slant on the forehead, the owner is more yang than yin. If the eyebrows are well-separated but curve downward, the owner is more yin than yang.

Long eyelashes are a yin characteristic. If the eyelids blink more often than once every 20 seconds, the person is far too yin. Frequent blinking is the eye's attempt, by action which is yang, to rid itself of surplus yin. Newborn babies, who are very yang, never blink.

The whole nervous system is involved when the eyes are enlarged. If the whites of the eyes are yellow or there are lines between the eyes, the liver's functioning is impaired. If the whites of the eyes are red or bloodshot, several disorders are indicated, depending upon the location of the redness on the surface of the eyeball.

The smaller the eyes, the stronger the constitution. Lines beneath the eyes denote a kidney ailment. A cancer patient will show blue in the whites of the eyes, but the face has a greenish cast.

Eyes reflect the body's change from yin to yang.

The ears are a measure of man's total condition. Normally, they extend from the eyes to the lower lip. But yin ears may reach farther because they are long and thin. Yang ears, shorter and higher, are more compact, much as the animals of the wild. A bird's ear can hear the smallest stirring of a worm in soft ground, yet it is so contracted, due to a yang diet of insects, worms and grain, that no outer structure

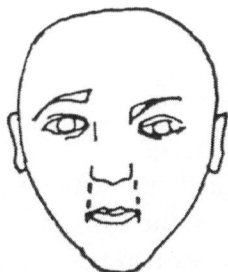

remains.

The width of the nose, nostril to nostril, should be the same width as the mouth. If the nose twists to the left, the father's constitution was stronger than the mother's; if it twists to the right, the mother's was stronger.

A yang nose is inclined to be compact with a tendency to flatness. A yin nose is pointed. If a woman, viewed head-on, has an almost geometrically straight nose, she is unable to bear children. The same nose on a man denotes homosexuality.

If the end of the nose is swollen, the heart is enlarged; a plane or plateau at the end of the nose denotes impaired cardiac functioning. Broken capillaries around the nose point to lung trouble.

The third area of the face, from the juncture of the nose and upper lip to the bottom of the chin, evidences the mold of the mother's nutriments during the last three months of pregnancy. The width of the mouth should be the same as the width of the nose. If the mouth is wider, the mother partook too freely of yin foods. The upper and lower lips should be of equal dimension. If the upper lip is enlarged or swollen, the stomach is expanded. If the lower lip is puffy or pendulous, there is distension in the large intestine. Yang lips are thin, neat, and well-defined. Dry, cracked, and peeling lips are a yang sign.

A protruding chin is a yin sign.

The teeth are the most yang part of the head. The lower jaw is regularly active in talking and chewing. If the teeth grow close together, they are normal. If there are gaps or separations (yin), a rift in the family is signaled for the near future. The yin physiological separation forecasts the societal one. A Chinese proverb says, "If teeth are split, he will not [be present to] see the death of his father," a grave offense in ancestor-conscious China.

Protruding teeth attests to yin attributes on the outside, yang on the inside. If only the lower teeth protrude, the person was well-endowed with yang properties at birth but thereafter ingested immoderate amounts of yin. Teeth that grow inward mark the presence of a high degree of yang.

Hand

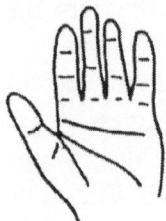

Palm up, divide the hand into three parts. Part 1, the fingers, reflects the condition of the nervous system. These extremities are the most yin. Part 2 reflects the circulation of the blood. Part 3, the inner area, reflects the state of the digestive organs and is the most yang part of the hand.

The lines of the hand reveal the history of the body's development. Strong, clean lines indicate natural healthy growth; broken, divided or multiple lines indicate the opposite. And when the growth and development were unsteady or uneven, that person's life has not been happy: When the physical is out of balance, thought and feeling suffer.

The first line below the fingers sketches one's emotional strength. If this line is uncertain or hesitant, the nervous system has developed erratically. If it is strong and clear, then consistent emotional health is a certainty. The line alongside the thumb between Part 2, the circulation, and Part 3, the digestive organs, shows the entire body strength and well-being.

Fingernails that are long or grow too fast, demonstrate a yin condition, as do fingernails that show white spots. The color of the nails should be pink; if it is a darker hue, or purple, then there has been an over-consumption of liquids, fruits, sugars, and the like. The angle between the thumb and index finger is a clue to the condition of the intestines. If this area is sensitive to manipulation, then constipation or other colonic disorder is present. Massage the area or tap it rhythmically several times a day with a round length of metal—a pen or pencil.

Yin-Yang Analysis
of Some Diseases

A. Albuminuria

This condition occurs when the Malpighian corpuscles, whose normal function is to filter salt and water, become dilated by excess yin and they begin to let albumin from the blood pass as well. It is rapidly cured by eliminating foods rich in sugar, potassium, and vitamin C and by eating more yang foods or simply a well-balanced diet.

B. Diabetes

Sugar is passed in the urine. Symptomatic medicine's answer is to give insulin and forbid the patient to eat anything rich in carbohydrates. This treatment ignores the cause, slows down the body processes, and reveals modern medicine's basic lack of understanding.

Ordinarily, Macrobiotic eating cures diabetes in several days. In rare cases, where the disease dates back 20 years or the cook is not too conscientious, the cure may take up to two or three months.

Sugar is yin and lack of insulin (which condenses sugar into a non-water-soluble sugar form) is also yin (the condenser being yang). Physically a very compact organ, the pancreas is yang. Functional incapacity of a yang organ is yin. Everywhere we find expansion—excess yin.

Well-balanced or slightly yang eating is recommended, as in the preliminary suggestions, and specifically: pumpkin, carrots, kuzu, buckwheat, gomasio, millet, and rice. Chew each mouthful 200 times.

C. Heart Disease

Why does the heart beat? What is the cause of this automatic body rhythm? No one knows. Modern medicine has no answer.

The unifying principle of yin and yang alone gives you the answer. If after studying the unifying principle, you still cannot answer these basic questions, then you won't be able to cure even varicose veins.

And if you cure yourself through the Macrobiotic way of eating and yet don't know why the heart beats, you are exclusive, selfish, arrogant, or unthankful. You will soon be sick or unhappy again.

Even doctors totally ignorant of the dialectic of yin/yang have succeeded in making artificial hearts and lungs for use during surgical operations. Billions of dollars spent in vain! 800,000 lives lost each year. Patients risking their lives for "scientific progress." Eighty-five percent success at Johns Hopkins where heart operations were performed while artificial organs replaced the original ones— 225 dead. At Children's Memorial Hospital in Chicago, Dr. Thomas Baffes transplanted the pulmonary artery and the aorta—15 out of 38 dead. What success! Great progress!

It seems that a wasteful, brutal force dominates Western thought and civilization. Capitalist mass production and mechanical inhuman distribution of goods make up Western world's economy. In the Orient, society's economy has been based on minimum consumption (vivere parvo), not abusing our infinite resources, even the moon's light! Production based on quality, beauty, and appreciation leads to total detachment and renunciation of material goods to reach independence, infinite freedom, and peace on earth. The East is the antithesis of the West in economics as well as in medicine.

Exaggerated *vivere parvo* becomes greed. Blind and mechanical imitation of a detached state makes you anyone's pawn. But abundant or surplus production and consumption removes the possibility of experiencing joyful and deep gratitude; they breed laziness and yin sicknesses because the worldly pleasures of such a society are yin by nature: heart disease, cerebral hemorrhage, cancer, kidney and liver disease, mental illness. [After heart disease and cancer, suicide is the third killer in the United States today.] Thousands of people awaiting surgery: frontal lobotomy, sympathectomy, heart, and kidney operations. The United States: 20th century hell!

Summary of Heart Diseases
Blue Baby:
Almost invariable signs are enlarged head, bulging eyes, bluish-white of the eyes, pug nose, lower lip larger than upper, flat feet, flat palms. All these show mother's extreme yin eating. She also may have similar physiological characteristics besides being selfish, arrogant, exclusive, unappreciative, or spoiled since her childhood: a real serpent.

Keeping such a deformed child or woman alive by bloody and totally artificial operations goes against the law of natural selection. But it holds the seeds of its own correction: the disintegration and the fall of the human race.

I have never seen a blue baby, but there must be a Macrobiotic cure. What has a beginning has an end. And if your understanding of justice (yin and yang) remains analytic and symptomatic, you will never enter the Kingdom of Heaven (Tao)!

Weak Heart:
According to Western medicine, it may be diagnosed through these symptoms.

1. As manifested in liver, lung, or kidney troubles: enlarged or painful liver, breathing difficulty, congestion, mucous discharge, oliguria, edema.

2. Cardio-vascular warnings (less dependable and shorter term than the more superficial symptoms): rapid heartbeat, blood pressure blockages, muffled heartbeat, heart murmur, irregular pulse, enlarged heart, irregular heartbeat.

3. First consider valvular imbalances, disorders of the aorta and

other principle arteries, congenital heart diseases. If possible, listen to the heartbeat with a stethoscope. Often you will have to wait for the spasm or contraction to reach its natural end.

4. If the blood pressure, especially the minimal, is very high, it may be a secondary form of Bright's disease (kidney) and an indication of heart failure.

5. Another patent cause, pulmonary sclerosis, aneurysm between an artery and a vein, swelling in one of the mitral or bicuspid valves, may be discovered in a routine examination.

6. If heart failure is apparently in an early stage, consider right away the possibility of adhesion between the parietal and visceral layers of the pericardium, rheumatism, failure of the myocardia (heart muscles), Basedow's disease (hyperthyroidism), heart strain, weak heart, coagulation in the myocardia, etc.

Treatment Typically Recommended by Occidental Medicine

1. Rest—absolute or partial bed rest.

2. Low salt or salt-free diet is prescribed in cases of swelling.

3. Treatment by surgery or other method is done to break any circulation blockages like serum-filled pockets, especially any pleural inflammations.

4. Treatment in the form of lancing and draining is done if cyanosis or high blood pressure is present.

5. After these treatments, a cathartic of German *eau de vie* and Nerprun syrup and theobromine is given for swelling, not to mention sedatives like morphine with digitalis or ouabain (glucoside from an African vegetable seed—local anaesthetic and a heart poison). Then treatment is done to the heart muscle itself.

   a. Digitalis is the standard drug for asystole with swelling and irregular heartbeat such as asystole of the mitral valve. It is contra-indicated in cases of extreme dilation of the heart chambers or rapid heartbeat, which in the case of acute asystole may precede sudden death.

   b. Ouabain by injection is the standard drug for failing left ventricles in hypertensive people. It is also used broadly in other kinds of asystole wherever digitalis is contra-indicated or ineffective. Sometimes it even sensitizes the heart to digitalis. Above all, it is an emergency drug; its action is short-term.

6. Additional means of heart stimulation include chemotherapy (drugs such as adonis, lily of the valley, spartein, strophantus, digitalis in minute amounts or ouabain in pill form. Vitamin B injections are given intravenously.

7. Theophylline is given when there is circulation impairment evidenced in electrocardiograms.

8. If the asystole is not relieved, the patient is prepared to tolerate a high dose of digitalis by taking graduated doses in increasing increments. Next, a mercurial diuretic is given such as novurit or neptal if the kidneys can withstand it (blood urea normal and urinations more or less normal). Also, anticoagulants are given to avoid thrombosis of the veins.

The Macrobiotic Interpretation of the Diagnosis

1. An enlarged or painful liver shows a really dangerous excess of yin. Breathing difficulty, congestion, and mucous discharge are all also yin, likewise oliguria and edema.

2. The cardio-vascular warnings are all symptoms of excessive yin eating.

3. Valvular imbalances, major arterial disorders, etc. show excessive yin present in the system.

4. High blood pressure caused by expansion is yin.

5. Sclerosis and hypertrophy of the cardiac walls are natural results of excess yin.

6. Symphysis of the pericardium is double yin: symphysis being caused by dilation and the pericardium being at the periphery (physical forms being yang at the center and yin at the surface). Because the nervous system has evolved from the ectoderm, all nervous diseases are yin, as are all skin conditions. Rheumatismal myocarditis is caused by excessive yin drinking. Basedow's disease by excessive potassium and vitamin C intake, also yin; so, also, are infarct and swelling.

Macrobiotic Critique of Orthodox Medicine's Treatment

1. Resting is yin. Enforced rest is death imposed by medicine operating on a sentimental level. Activity is life. Yin-eating produces yin sickness, incapacitating (yinnizing) the motor activity of all the body's organs. First we must eliminate yin elements from the body. But complete immobility hinders this elimination and so weakens the heart even more. Organs like all living tissues function well only with repeated exercising (expanding and contracting).

2. A salt-free diet is extremely yin. To yinnize such patients even further is fatal; I don't understand such sensory judgment. In Europe, everywhere, I have seen only aggravation of such conditions caused by lack of salt, which, continued a year or more, leads to total exhaustion. Why this salt phobia? The child who renounces his very blood can only suffer perpetual fear.

3. Break circulation blockages?—childish thinking, symptomatic. Why not get to the source?

4. Lance and drain cyanosis?—primitive brutality. You must understand that the quality of the blood determines the organ's health and that the way of eating can radically change organs.

5. German *eau de vie* and Nerprun are both extremely yin, as are theobromine, morphine, and ouabain. Only digitalis is relatively yang. Great yin repels and hides smaller yin. What kind of cure replaces lesser sickness with a more extreme one? Isn't it curious that we know by trial and error not to use digitalis in cases of acute enlargement of the heart or possible severe asystole? Know-how without conceptual understanding is lethal. Western medicine is not scientific; Eastern science is rooted in a whole-universe view. They separate the relative from the absolute, the infinite and the eternal. Western science, even the natural sciences, knows only the relative world, the physical evolving finite world.

6. How contradictory—symptomatic empirical medicine! Adonis and lily of the valley are very yang whereas strophanthus and sparteine (especially in the form of sulfates, campho-carbonates, or campho-sulfonates) are very yin. Without the unifying principle of yin and yang, there is no compass. How tragic!

7 & 8. Likewise. Naturally anything which inhibits coagulation (▲) is yin (▼).

Use the dialectic of yin and yang to arrive at a Macrobiotic treatment: practical and extremely simple. The heart being among the most yang organs is especially vulnerable to excess yin. Elimination of this excess is the only secret behind miracle heart condition cures.

Angina Pectoris: (Ninety percent fatal over a 20-year period)

Occidental diagnosis —

1. Shows up under strain or during the night when the patient is in a reclining position.

2. Painful constriction in the heart.

3. Acute attacks leading to sudden death, myocardiac infarct, failure of the left ventricle.

Symptomatic occidental treatment—During the attack, amyl nitrite, or better, trinitrine. At other times, look for syphilitic aortitis, failure of the left ventricle. Prescribe health foods; avoid rich foods and overeating, walking after meals and exposure to cold. Shortwave therapy, novocaine, thermal cures. Surgical operation: sympathectomy.

Dialectic Macrobiotic Treatment

Angina pectoris attacks people who have eaten much yin food in a relatively short time. Here are a couple of case histories typical among Macrobiotic people.

A Japanese doctor, age 52, who was petrified at the idea of intravenous feeding, followed the Macrobiotic way of eating after many years of heart trouble. A few weeks later, he was up gardening at the break of dawn and has since spent several years as my assistant.

One of Japan's most respected doctors, age 81, whose well-equipped office was located in the big industrial city of Osaka, became disillusioned with Western medicine because he was unable to cure his only son. Despite pleas from his many renowned colleagues, he had taken up the co-directorship of a hospital in Kyoto famous for its unorthodox and highly imaginative approach to the sickness that had taken his only son's life. There he stumbled onto one of my books and afterwards came with his wife—both of them in traditional dress—to visit me in my Tokyo clinic. With great ceremonial humility, he asked simply to study *in vivo* with me. Three years later, he returned to his native country armed with a firm grasp of the Unifying Principle and accompanied by his wife who had mastered the high art of cooking. They write:

> How can we thank you for your deep and invaluable teaching! We are very happy. For the first time, we understand the true meaning of medicine and the nature of sickness. Now I am free to ask my son's forgiveness for my complete ignorance.

The day he left, dressed as on that first day in his samurai habit, tears came to his eyes. Now, 17 years later, I still see them occasionally in my dreams, impeccable in their deep sense of order, totally unassuming in their faithfulness.

Irregular Heartbeat:
Symptomatic diagnosis, as usual, is superficial, groping, palliative, violent, traumatic, and above all, unscientific. Quinidine gives a 50 percent chance of being cured; and so, a 50 percent chance of failure!

The preliminary diet brings such quick and easy relief.

Acute Rapid Heartbeat:
Although symptomatic medicine says only five percent die of this disease, it offers no cure, only a life sentence to heart condition. Besides breathing exercises and a low-fat diet that the patient usually arrives at intuitively, occidental symptomatic medicine suggests:

1. Rest
2. Induce vomiting.
3. Give intravenous feeding of quinidine.
4. If the above are ineffective, prescribe novocaine.

Macrobiotic treatment is all too easy and accessible to anyone: preliminary diet with one or two teaspoons of gomasio at meals.

Chronic slow pulse, according to symptomatic medicine, may become acute at any moment. In fact, says macrobiotic understanding, there exist two kinds: the yin and the yang slow pulse. The yang variety poses no threat. But the yin is very serious. Stick to the preliminary diet for a couple of weeks with rice cream and one large umeboshi daily. I know of a case where a Catholic priest was cured of this condition after one acupuncture session. The cure could not last, however, because he was too attached to analytic dualistic thinking to accept the dialectic tool of yin and yang.

Rheumatic Heart:

According to symptomatic medicine, rheumatism is at the base of 95 percent of valvular heart conditions. It is a progressive disease in that it leads to death in 66 percent of its cases. A cobbler could do better than that! You'd be safer at the flea market than in the hospital. Try the Macrobiotic way of eating.

Standard treatment for heart trouble consists simply in eating well-cooked rice cream, buckwheat cream, or rolled oats. "Incurable" does not exist in the macrobiotic vocabulary. Quite honestly, symptomatic medicine admits it has no real cure for this number one killer. Its dietary prescriptions, like its drugs, are sentimental and fall helter-skelter along the yin/yang continuum. [1973, USA: Heart disease is called the number one killer—scapegoat for our ignorance. Cancer is number two—tumors of our excess, physical, mental and spiritual baggage. Suicide is number three—another form of genocide and war.]

Well, what is the heart? It is the body's rhythm-maker. Its health is dependent on the quality and quantity of the blood. Yin blood rushes to the yang heart; yang blood runs to the yin periphery. On its way, it picks up oxygen in the lungs and drops off wastes in the kidneys. So, in fact, the blood pumps the heart. The heart's strength comes from the blood's ability to change, to transmute, to reverse its yin/yang polarity.

You ask: How do we stop and regain life? How to flow with change? How to initiate change? For the heart: change blood quality by good eating and regain memory by long chewing. For cancer: eat and fast; *vivere parvo*. For the schizophrenic insanity that leads to war, genocide, and suicide: share and understand that what you eat is as much for the happiness and health of the people around you, your ancestors, and children to come, as for your own. Pray actively.

D. Hyperthyroidism
Symptomatic medicine cuts out part or all of this vital endocrine gland, sometimes with apparent success, sometimes with utter failure. Two or three months of macrobiotic eating should completely transform a person suffering from this condition.

Without the tool of yin and yang, symptomatic medicine cannot progress beyond categorizing and symptom-chasing with the devastating results that great yin repelling little yin must lead to new diseases—iatrogenic diseases.

E. Deformed Bodies and Spirits
Giving birth to a deformed child (harelip, hydrocephalic, encephalic, ophthalmic, sexually abnormal, blue baby, etc.) means a lifetime of suffering and regret, especially if your child is mentally retarded, mongoloid, or deaf-mute.

Birth defects, both physical and psychological, are increasing rather than decreasing today. In the United States, the yearly number of blue babies is estimated between 30,000 and 80,000. There is probably a total of more than a million birth defects—children destined to a lifetime of mediocre suffering. But beware: if you're living under the illusion that chronic sickness and unhappiness are as incurable as hereditary disease, then you will suffer as much as a congenitally-ill person. In fact, birth defects are often not as sad as progressive, degenerative, or acute sicknesses.

In Brussels, I met a 66-year-old woman who for 13 years had been suffering from excess sexual desire. An operation 14 years before followed 20 earlier years of sickness. Her suffering was deeper than that of many congenitally-sick people.

According to Macrobiotic medicine, all homosexuality and hermaphrodism should be considered very serious sicknesses—as much a part of society's involvement as of the person himself. Sexual pathology, like color-blindness is far more prevalent in the West than in the East.

The female man and the male woman are not uncommon today. The really strong, brave, daring, and imaginatively energetic man is rare. Rare, also, is the soft delicate woman, biding, slow to anger, and quick to bend. Few women understand how to contain the yang within and remain yin on the outside. Everywhere petty quarrels: yang rebuffing yang; yin repelling yin. People exteriorize their yang as violence and crudeness.

Rough-skinned women with much body hair, mustaches, irregular painful and excessive periods are already sexually sick. So, also, are the effeminate men with no deep sense of daring or of justice—personal or social. Cotton-candy men!

What is the deep cause of so many birth defects? What is at the root of all this sexual pathology?

Sentimental indulgence in eating without any overall understanding: man's original fall from Eden. Gone is the strong-hearted clear vision—exchanged for plastic food, gluttony, turning to doctors for symptomatic relief and overnight panaceas, antibiotics, hormone therapy, cortisone, x-rays, vaccinations, inoculations, radium treatments.

There you have it: the "miracle" cures are the most recent cause of the disease, suffering, and killing that surround us and haunt us.

Among research scientists, the dangers of exposure to x-rays is well known. Between 1905 and 1938, various experiments with x-rays led to documented cases of cataracts, club feet, and toeless feet in guinea pigs. The longer and the more intense the exposure to x-rays, the more severe the birth defects are.

In 1920, Aschenheim noted the birth of a baby with an undersized brain and malformed eyes where the mother had received radium treatment of the uterus during her first four months of pregnancy.

By 1926, Zapper had collected 20 case histories of externally provoked birth defects. A year later, Goldstein and Murphy found 37.3 percent of a random group of mothers exposed to x-rays gave birth to children with physiological or psychological anomalies.

Hale (1935) raised piglets with cleft palates, harelips, kidney malfunctions, eye defects—all originating from the lack of vitamin A during early pregnancy. Warkany and Schrafenberger (1944) bred rats, 30 percent of them with physiological abnormalities correlated with vitamin B_2 deficiencies in the mothers. An understanding of the yin and yang of vitamins and of pigs and rats will reveal to you a clearer interpretation of their conclusion.

Hormonal imbalances and excesses cause birth defects. Fraser (1935) experimenting with mice and rabbits found cortisone injections intimately connected with cleft palates, similarly with the introduction of 17 hydroxycorticosterone and ACTH.

Giving surplus insulin to birds and perhaps mammals as well raises the probability of freak mutations. Similarly in man, diabetes or predisposition to diabetes leads to congenital diseases in the offspring.

There is a clear time-correlation between the introduction of excess vitamin A in the mother and the development of deformed organs and malfunctions in the fetus.

All these observations show that the causes of birth defects are most potent during the earliest stages of morphogenesis. The embryo is most vulnerable in its first fifteen days; that is, the time preceding organ formation. The month-and-a-half immediately following reveals increased sensitivity; malformations are actually produced that never totally disappear, at least from the nervous system.

The causes of these malformations may be slight in themselves.

"Mongolism has been clearly demonstrated to be a function of genetic factors; its frequency increases with the mother's age (Turpin, 1934, and Shroder 1939)."

Actually, the mother's age is not the key. Often a woman tends to lead a softer life as she ages, eating more yin foods, pastries, fruit, imported delicacies, yin drinks. Naturally she spoils her children with what she herself desires—yin. Children brought up by grand-parents are even more yin (age brings a natural dehydration which craves yin). Retirement and a higher percentage of vegetables and fruits in their diet is the expected reaction to the more active meat-eating days of their youth. An old Japanese saying goes: The child raised without a father will lack will in his life; his sense of virtue and justice will be diminished by 50 percent; the child brought up by the grandmother will go crazy, his sense of justice diminished by 70 percent. So we interpolate that the child raised by his mother and grandmother loses 100 percent of his love of justice.

Conclusion:

I am continually shocked and saddened by the widespread sexu-al aberrances and birth defects in the West. And occidental medicine by its own confession is completely ignorant of possible causes and cures. Medical research scientists and doctors alike are helpless to heal even their own bodies. They do not look beyond the immediate outward appearances.

So many churches and holy days! Saints galore. Every Sunday, church on TV. God created in the image of man. Barbaric super-stition. Empty ritual. A zombie world seeking flash gratification, speeding towards a tragic end. Psychotic fear and alienation from self, from others.

Ask (for the ability to really enjoy and express gratitude) and it shall be given unto you; seek (true justice) and ye shall find it (it has never been taken away—you had it all the while). You, man-kind, have just forgotten and moved away. What the world seeks now is gold, power, fame, know-how, and techniques. So it finds just that: a multitude of possible causes of congenital diseases—physi-cal, chemical, drug induced, iatrogenic, vitamin deficiencies, germs, viruses that leave in their tracks even greater sicknesses. We forget that physiological sicknesses and even more psychological prob-lems stem from the food we feed on, our external environment, in its broadest sense.

What stands in our way?

1. Our loss of memory and poor judgment [the origin of our sickness and unhappiness].

2. Our facile conceptual understanding (yin) fools us and paralyzes us; we lack the slow willful doing, the long sure application (yang).

But we do know that everything changes into its opposite. The yin/yang compass guides us smoothly out of the throes of our impasse. The great tragedy for me is seeing how far the 20th century has strayed from simple traditional eating and frenetically seeks satisfaction from what can never satisfy or even satiate it.

F. Warts and Skin Growths

We disregard warts or dismiss them as irrelevant. In fact, they are not only annoying and ugly but a sign of excess animal protein. A woman with warts rarely becomes happy even if she is otherwise bright, attractive, and wealthy.

Warts reveal greed and selfishness. Because it takes seven times more land to raise animals than grains for human consumption, over-eating animal-quality food represents a real social crime. It inevitably leads to hardening of the arteries, arthritis, rheumatism, facial paralysis, miscarriages or sterility, unfaithful mates or children.

Symptomatic medicine has no real cure for warts but instead cuts or burns them out. New ones spring up. Isn't violence used in medical treatment a cover-up for ignorance?

Once I treated a girl who had 200 warts, some as big as chestnuts, others the size of soybeans. She had been adopted by a very yang midwife; she was hostile and exuded a real stench. During the first few weeks of her cure, the warts started to shrivel. At the end of three months, they had all fallen off by themselves. The strong odor had disappeared, and the girl was radiant.

Then, curiously, a couple of new ones started growing; the girl had sneaked a few fried shrimp. Proof enough that what we eat becomes our blood and creates our karma, both physical and psychological.

Symptomatic medicine sees warts, corns, callouses, planters' warts, and other skin excrescences as the result of continual pressure or rubbing, hereditary factors, secondary developments of venereal diseases, some primitive lichen-like fungi-innumerable Latin terms—but no cure. Treatments given: surgical removal, burning with fire or acid, electrolysis, exposure to ultraviolet light—all violent means that only destroy the natural warning signs, the body's indictment of our piggishness and selfishness.

Sickness and Foods

No sickness can be completely cured without following
the way of eating according to the order of nature.

– Caraka Samhita

Establishing infinite freedom, eternal happiness and absolute integrity (justice) without artifice or violence: This is
my practical philosophy.

– Lao-tse

Macrobiotic medicine is nothing but a biological and dialectic application of the highest philosophy of the Far
East, the matrix of the civilization and all the great religions of the East, including Christianity, Hinduism, Brah-
manism, Islam and Buddhism. Acupuncture, moxibustion
and massage as well as the pharmaceutical medicine of
China and India belong to the earliest and most primitive stage of oriental medicine. Its highest development is
macrobiotics and the way of eating.

– George Ohsawa

Achieve yin/yang balance in the composition, proportion, and preparation of your daily food.

A change in the kitchen changes the chemistry of life. It is as
simple as that.

Your food is transformed; it becomes flesh and blood, becomes
feelings, impulses, emotions, thoughts, actions, love, hate.

Change the quality of the brain and nervous system (blood, tissue, cells) to cure mental illness.

The Unique Principle—pure and perfect law of the universe—will strike the chord of pure and perfect principle in you, and thus evoke the celestial harmony of inner accord.

One's physical and psychological condition depends upon the proportion and preparation of the food one eats. The yin/yang proportion must always be 5 to 1.

The medicine that cures once and forever is the medicine based upon justice, as Ruskin outlines in *Unto This Last* (*Philosophy of Oriental Medicine*, page 6).

According to Alexis Carrel, disease has two classes—infectious or microbian diseases, and degenerative diseases. Infectious diseases are caused by viruses or bacteria penetrating into the body. However, in many people they remain inoffensive.

Carrel said in the book *Man, The Unknown*:

> Among human beings, some are subject to disease and others are immune. Such a state of resistance is due to the individual constitution of the tissues and the humors which oppose the penetration of pathogenic agents or destroy them when they have invaded our body. This is natural immunity. This form of immunity may preserve certain individuals from almost any disease. It is one of the most precious qualities for which man could wish. We are still ignorant of its nature.

According to Chinese medicine, human immunity depends on the quality of blood, especially of red cells and white cells. In other words, if we have healthy blood, we will be immune from any infectious disease. How can we make blood healthy? I leave this question for awhile—and I go on about the degenerative diseases that are caused, according to Carrel, by certain disorders such as the deficiency of endocrine secretion, gastric mucosa, etc.

> The deficiency of endocrine glands, of thyroid, pancreas, liver, and gastric mucosa, brings on diseases such as myx-

edema, diabetes, pernicious anemia, etc. Other disorders are determined by the absence of elements required for the construction and maintenance of tissues, such as vitamins, minerals, salts, iodine, and metals. When organs do not receive from the cosmic world, through the intestine, the building substances they need, they lose their power of resistance to infection, develop structural lesions, manufacture poison, etc. There are also diseases that have so far baffled all the scientists and the institutes for medical research of America, Europe, Africa, Asia, and Australia. Among them are cancer and a multitude of nervous and mental afflictions.

From the macrobiotic viewpoint, degenerative diseases result from the shortage or excess of required elements for the construction and maintenance of tissues, organs, and the nervous system, such as vitamins, mineral salts, and enzymes. This, in short, is the result of ill blood cells that build ill organs. According to Dr. K. Chishima and Dr. K. Morishita, blood cells are produced through digested food in the intestine wall, contrary to the normal medical belief that blood is produced in bone marrow.

Dr. K. Chishima wrote in his newly published book, *Revolution of Biology and Medicine*, Vol. 9:

> According to my opinion the red blood corpuscles in higher animals are a basal element from which almost all kinds of cells are derived, while there can be found no firm evidence that red blood corpuscles proliferate in the normal bone marrow. The author agrees with opinion presented by Duran-Jorda (1947-1951) who claims that the bone marrow of high animals is not a site of red blood cell production but red blood corpuscles are produced within the granular leucocyte in the intestinal wall.

He claims that cells also originate from blood:

> The origin of the primordial germ cells has been studied by

Swift (1915), Brode (1928), Dantschakoff (1931), Matsumoto (1931), Goldsmith (1928) and many other scientists. But as all of these investigators are believers of orthodox cell theory, ever since Virchow, their opinion regarding the origin of germ cells differs with facts on certain important points. I have studied about this problem on chick embryos, at the Laboratory of Zootechnical Science, Kyushu Imperial University, and I have found that the primordial germ cells of chicks arise at first on the blood island (outer side of embryo), by means of new formation of cells from yolk spheres, but not by mitotic cell division. In other words, the germ cells and other cellular elements of gonads are the derivatives from differentiated red corpuscles.

Also, according to Dr. Chishima, normal protoplasm transforms into pathological protoplasm, pathological bacteria, and viruses. If this is the case, immunity is nothing but an ability to prevent this pathological transformation. In short, immunity or prevention of degenerative disease is dependent on good blood, then on good food. On this point, Alexis Carrel warned us about the importance of food more than 30 years ago in *Man, The Unknown*.

The effect of the chemical compounds contained in food upon physiological and mental activities is far from being thoroughly known. Medical opinion on this point is of little value, for no experiments of sufficient duration have been made upon human beings to ascertain the influence of a given diet. There is no doubt that consciousness is affected by the quantity and the quality of the food. We have to discover, which food is suitable for human beings vegetating in offices and factories. Which chemical substances could give intelligence, courage, and alertness to the inhabitants of the new city. The race will certainly not be improved merely by supplying children and adolescents with a great abundance of milk, cream, and all known vitamins. It would be most useful to search for new compounds that instead of use-lessly increasing the size and weight of the skeleton and of the muscles, would bring about nervous strength and mental agility.

Right Foods

Before we discuss the Macrobiotic diet, we have to know what is the right food for man. *The Yearbook of Agriculture, 1959–Food*, published by The United States Department of Agriculture, is a good source of information on modern nutrition. It shows "Recommended Daily Dietary Allowances," on pages 228 and 229. (See chart next page.)

These are the daily dietary nutrients recommended by United States authority. However, there are several questions on this.

Q1. If these nutrients are recommended to maintain good health, then what is the definition of health?

Weight, height, and strength of muscle is not enough to measure health.

Q2. What is the source of calories?

According to the "Yearbook," ice cream, milk, grains, fat, etc. are all the same source of calories. However, from my experiences, ice cream and grains are entirely different sources of calories. If we eat only ice cream to supply 3,000 calories a day, we will become insane! Also, whole grains and refined grains are different sources of calories. Analytical nutritional theory is not analytical enough in this point.

Q3. What is the better source of protein?

The modern nutritional theory recommends animal protein rath-

Recommended Daily Dietary Allowances By The U.S. Department of Agriculture
The Yearbook of Agriculture 1959

	Age Yrs.	Wt. Lbs.	Ht. In.	Calories	Pro-tein Gm.	Cal-cium Gm.	Iron Mg.	Vit. A I.U.	Thia-mine Mg.	Ribo-flavin Mg.	Niacin equiv. Mg.	Vit. C	Vit. D
Men	25	154	69	3,200	70	.8	10	5,000	1.6	1.8	21	75	—
	45	154	69	3,000	70	.8	10	5,000	1.5	1.8	20	75	—
	65	154	69	2,550	70	.8	10	5,000	1.3	1.8	18	75	—
Women	25	128	64	2,300	58	.8	12	5,000	1.2	1.5	17	70	—
	45	128	64	2,200	58	.8	12	5,000	1.1	1.5	17	70	—
	65	128	64	1,800	58	.8	12	5,000	1.0	1.5	17	70	—
Pregnant (second half)				+300	+20	1.5	15	6,000	1.3	2.0	+3	100	400
Lactating (28 oz. daily)				+1,000	+40	2.0	15	8,000	1.7	2.5	+2	150	400
Infant in mos.	2-6	13	24	lb.x54.5	(1)	.6	5	1,500	.4	.5	6	30	400
	7-12	20	28	lb.x45.4	(1)	.8	7	1,500	.5	.8	7	30	400
Children	1-3	27	34	1,300	40	1.0	7	2,000	.7	1.0	8	35	400
	4-6	40	43	1,700	50	1.0	8	2,500	.9	1.3	11	50	400
	7-9	60	51	2,100	60	1.0	10	3,500	1.1	1.5	14	60	400
	10-12	79	57	2,500	70	1.2	12	4,500	1.3	1.8	17	75	400
Boys	13-15	108	64	3,100	85	1.4	15	5,000	1.6	2.1	21	90	400
	16-19	139	69	3,600	100	1.4	15	5,000	1.8	2.5	25	100	400
Girls	13-15	108	63	2,600	80	1.3	15	5,000	1.3	2.0	17	80	400
	16-19	120	64	2,400	75	1.3	15	5,000	1.2	1.9	16	80	400

(1) Allowances are not given for protein during infancy, but intakes of 1.5 grams of protein for each pound of body weight are ample for healthy infants.

er than vegetable protein because the former has balanced amino acids. However, many scholars are against animal foods.

(Please read *Macrobiotics: An Invitation to Health and Happiness*, by George Ohsawa, *Are You Confused*, by Paavo Airola, and *Food is Your Best Medicine*, by Dr. Henry Beiler, etc.)

Q4. What about milk as a source of calcium?

As the source of calcium, the book recommends milk. However, milk is not a food for man. Future scientific study will reveal that cow's milk lacks the proper nutrition for the development of the brain in man.

Q5. What is the best source of iron?
Q6. What is the best source of vitamins?

Modern nutrition strongly recommends vitamins, especially vitamin C. However, this requirement is the result of meat-eating. For vegetarians, this requirement will be different. Whole grains and vegetables will supply enough vitamins without fruits.

Q7. If this recommendation is agreed upon, how do we know we are getting those nutrients without chemical analysis?

We may be able to calculate the food nutrients using the food value table. However, the table shows only an average of the value that certain foods have. The individual foods you are going to eat will have different values than mentioned in the table. For example, any orange will contain different amounts of vitamin C depending on when and how it is grown, how it is cultivated, stored, delivered, etc. The older one will have less vitamin C than the fresher one.

In other words, the table is static, but reality is dynamic and everything is always changing. Therefore, such a food table has not much value from the practical point of view.

There are many books and magazines in this country, like Dr. Walker's book, *Diet and Salad Suggestion*. Some of them are best sellers, as for example, *Folk Medicine* and *Prevention* magazine. All of them are empirical, and authors endeavor to generalize individual experiences. However, they do not have a basic principle and lack an understanding of life, health, freedom, happiness, and integrity (justice), the primordial things in this world. And because they lack any basic understanding of the order, balance, and functioning of the universe and of man, their knowledge, techniques, ideologies, and prescriptions are at best superstitious and at worst dangerous and criminal.

When one is equipped with the unique principle of Oriental philosophy—the eyeglasses of yin/yang—one can see the danger of such empirical, individual, and analytical knowledge and the anarchic application of such knowledge. The implications are, in fact, appalling. But modern man is very primitive, simple, and extremely near-sighted. He is convinced very easily by these publications with their long, lucid, scientific explanations. Simple man surrenders to anything complex. This is the inferiority complex of the masses.

Modern occidental science is very complicated in its appearance, but in reality it is extraordinarily simple and rigid in its theory. Furthermore, it is destructive because it is analytical rather than integrative, and microscopic rather than panoramic and total in its point of view. But simple man, who cannot think and judge for himself, surrenders before any power, commercial, economic, or intellectual. Thus, the modern occidental world is full of superstitions, just as in the Middle Ages or in primitive tribes. The only difference between modern and medieval superstition is the difference between complexity and mysticism.

Pasteurization, for example, which is generally accepted nowadays, is a form of modern superstition. There are superstitions, however, that are far more dangerous and the cause of the pandemic diseases that plague modern man; the so-called superiority of animal protein, and the notion that sugar, fruit juice, and milk are proper foods for man. Although in other areas Dr. Walker's book is full of serious errors, his scientific reasoning against the use of milk is sound and convincing.

It must be remembered that scientific knowledge has never been able to establish human happiness, health, and freedom. In Biblical times, the scientists (scribes) were rejected by Jesus along with the hypocritical Pharisees. In the last 50 years, medical knowledge has increased a hundredfold more than in the 2,500 years since Hippocrates. And yet, the state of human health has worsened to such an extent that "medicine men," including specialists, are now desperately crying out for a "God only knows" medicine. This state of affairs is documented in *Time* magazine, March 7, 1960 and *Realités*, February 1960 (a French magazine).

Macrobiotics has an entirely different way of considering the diet and nutrition. It considers first—What is man? What is the Order of Nature? and What are the principles that govern the life of man and animals? etc. Without answering those questions, there will be no right answers to What are man's right foods? It is, therefore, understandable that there is so much controversy in health diets today.

A. What is Man?

In order to know the right foods for man, we must know what is man. From whence does your body come? Where was your body 10 months before your birth? The hen comes from an egg, and the egg comes from a hen. "There are some riddles impossible to solve, such as whether the hen or the egg came first" said the greatest philosopher of modern France, H. Bergson. There are many questions of this kind. All of these enigmatic questions are amusing like "Columbus' Egg," and the famous "Seven Enigmas of the Universe" of Du Bois Reymond and are good to strengthen our judgment toward the goal of Supreme judging ability. Let us uncover our highest judging ability!

I asked this question to the audience at my lectures at the Buddhist Academy during this winter. A student answered, "We came from the food that we are taking daily." What a wonderful answer it is. I gave him the highest honor, because his judging ability had cleared so much. What food is the origin of the whole animal kingdom? The vegetal world. Even the animals that feed themselves on lower animals, ultimately depend upon vegetables.

An important discovery of modern occidental physiology tells us, to our amazement, what had been discovered some thousands of years ago in the Orient: Only vegetables can assimilate inorganic matter and produce organic substances such as carbohydrates, protein, or fat. Another discovery (heterotropism) tells us that animals destroy these products of autotropism to make their own physiological construction and dynamic energy. Thousands and thousands of years ago, all great religions of the East knew this and taught mankind to eat 100 percent cereals and vegetables to lead man towards the Kingdom of Happiness.

Starting from these facts (autotropism and heterotropism), we must deduce that the vegetal kingdom is the mother of animals and the staple food for the construction of the human body, while animal foods are secondary. But occidental logic, backbone of all the Western civilization (Kantian logic), deduces that animal foods are more useful and convenient to human body construction. This was produced and experimented with very superficially by Liebig in the beginning of the 19th century. He stressed the importance of animal protein and fat. Kantian logic and its physiological counterpart—Liebig's theory of animal nutrition for man—is the very antipode of the Eastern (Vedantic) philosophy and its physiological technique.

Vegetable foods are all grasses, leaves, stems, roots, flowers, and seeds (grains). We are nothing but a transformation of grasses. The Japanese word corresponding to grass is "Kusa." (Kusa in Sanskirt means sacred grass.) There is a universal worship of "Kusa," the sacred grass. Since the very beginning of Japan, the biggest ceremony in Japan is the Emperor's ceremony of "Kusa" when he ascends the throne. The highest Shintoist shrine of Japan is Geguh Ise, where the Goddess Toyouke is worshipped. The Goddess has another name: Uka-no-Mitama. This means: She is the producer of all "Kusa," or sacred grass; rice, wheat, millet, and other grains are nothing but the incarnation of the Goddess Toyouke, the Principle of Life. There are hundreds of thousands of shrines. Inari (producer of "Ine" or "Uruchi," the Japanese version of the Sanskrit word "Wrch" representing rice), is another popular name of Toyouke. The sacred grass signifies the most important, universal foods. National worship of this Principle of Life is the most traditional and important cult of Japan.

But what is the origin of this vegetal world?

The earth, mother of all life, is a huge mass of inorganic elements producing all kinds of organic forms. If it is said that man is made of dust (earth) in the Bible, then it is literally correct and can even be justified by modern biology and physiology. "Earth or dust" means all chemical elements, including the components air and water. According to modem science, some 100 elements are known. (According to our philosophy, there are at least 256 elements.)

What is the origin of the earth, the elements?

The origin of the elements is the "pre-atomic" or fourth "heaven." (Some of them have been discovered by modern science such as the electron, proton, positron, neutron, neutrino, photon, etc.)

From whence does this pre-atomic realm come?

It is certain that they are the products of energy.

What is the origin of energy?

It is very simple: two antagonistic poles, Yin and Yang (In and Yo in Japanese) produce energy—the sixth "heaven."

Where do these two poles come from?

Two must come from One, the infinite, eternal, and absolute Oneness, the Universe, the Wholeness, the Wholesomeness, the Holiness, or Seventh Heaven.

If you start from the Oneness going down towards man, this is the story of Genesis. You will be able to justify Genesis and find a new interpretation of the theory of evolution.

The world of man (the first) is very yang (noisy, rushing, conflicting, killing, destroying). The second or vegetable kingdom, on the contrary, is yin (quiet, nonmovement, no red blood). But the third world, the earth, is yang. It is rotating and revolving at a great speed, while the fourth world, or pre-atomic, is again yin, noiseless and colorless. The fifth world of energy is yang, as it is energetic and dynamic. It is the generator of all the activities and ceaseless changing in this world. The sixth world of two poles must be static and yin. Thus, starting from the animal kingdom (yang), we arrived at the sixth world of two static poles via four worlds, yin-yang-yin-yang. The higher realm is the origin of the next smaller numbered world. Here is the chart of our universe, the Key of the Infinite, Eternal, and Absolute, including six finite, changing, determinate, and immediate worlds in spiralic form. This is the mandala of the conception—constitution of the universe showing the origin of man, vegetables, minerals, pre-atoms, energy, and two poles, respectively. More minutely speaking, the constitution of our universe is a huge logarithmic spiral.

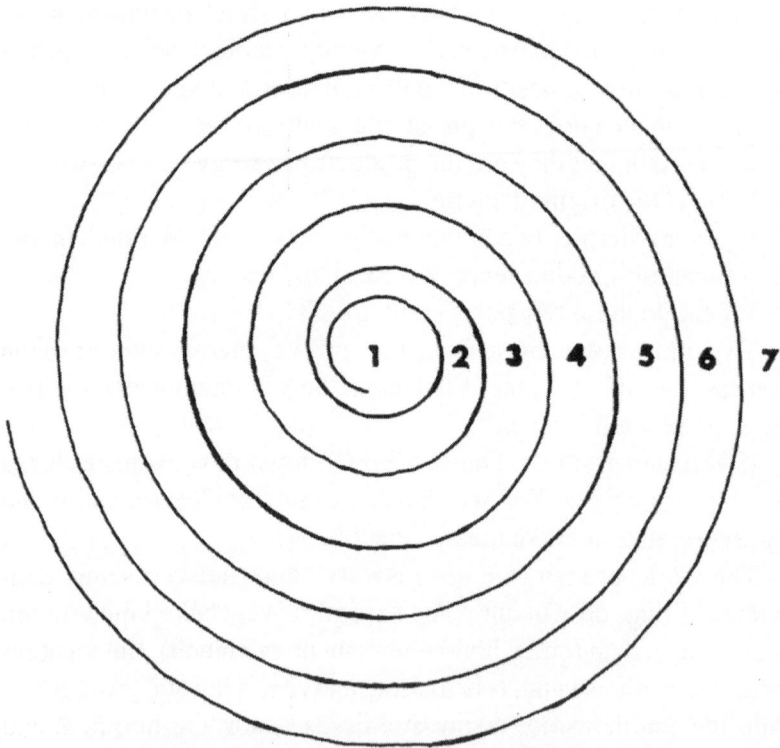

1. Animal (Hemoglobin)   2. Vegetal (Plant)   3. Element (Earth)   4. Pre-atomic
5. Energy   6. Two Poles   7. Oneness (External World)

INFINITY

INFINITY

INFINITY

Relative World
Visible World

MATERIALISTIC, REALISTIC, PHENOMENAL
AND INDIVIDUAL WORLD
BODY DESIRE, BIG AND SMALL, STRONG
AND WEAK, POSITIVE AND NEGATIVE,
PARA-SYMPATHETIC AND SYMPATHETIC

TIME
SPACE
SENSORY
KNOWLEDGE
TECHNIQUE

INFINITY WORLD

SPIRIT, ABSOLUTE, DREAM,
INVISIBLE WORLD, WONDERLAND
TRUTH, ETERNITY, LIBERTY,
METAPHYSICAL WORLD

The order from the first to the sixth world of "Heaven" is the very Order of the Universe. This Order of the Universe is the only dominant principle of the relative world. Yin produces yang, and yang produces yin, and so on forever. This is the foundation of the Oriental, Vedantic logic. That is so practical and so convenient that one can use it at the same time in the six finite and inconstant worlds of relativity and in the infinite, absolute, and eternal universe—that is to say, in the world of matter and in the world of spirit. Western logic is limited in its validity to the first six worlds and quite useless in the spiritual universe—the seventh heaven.

The chaos and tragedy of man is due to the abuse of this formal logic in the absolute, infinite, eternal, and indeterminate universe of spirituality and to neglect of the difference between the finite and the infinite.

Life is an infinite flux of energy; a part of its passage is called

"Man," and another "Vegetables," "Elements," and "Pre-Atoms" are other parts of the same flux. The elements, or the inorganic world, give themselves to become the vegetables, the vegetables give themselves to become man.

Because Fig. 1, "The Spiral of Life," is a continuous spiral, there are no separations between Animal-Plant-Element-Pre-Atom-Energy-Two Poles-Oneness in reality, although to our sensorial perception they are separate entities. Here is an origin of dualism and dichotomy, that is to say, the separation of Man and Nature, the separation of Body and Mind.

Furthermore, this spiral tells us the important fact that the seventh world, oneness, Eternal One, God, is the producer or the origin of the sixth to the first worlds. The sixth world of two poles, yin and yang, is the producer or the origin of the fifth to the first worlds. In the same token, the vegetal world (the second) is the producer or the origin of the animal world, including man.

An understanding of this Order of the Universe brings us to the first principle of foods for man. Man's life is directly dependent on the vegetal world. In other words, man's right foods are basically vegetables (this includes grains). In the temperate zone, man's food should consist of about seven times more vegetables than animal foods, or you can even eliminate animal foods completely if you use the proper amounts of salt and condiments in cooking. (This ratio derived from the fact that man has four canine teeth used for cutting animal foods, and 28 teeth, used for chewing grains and vegetables. Also, the K/Na ratio in the blood plasma is about 7 to 1. Because K represents the vegetal world and Na represents the animal world, this ratio can be written as K/Na as vegetable/animal—7/1.)

However, man is free. He can eat as much animal foods as he wants. If, however, he continues such a diet for a long time, he will reach a point where his body cannot maintain a proper balance of yin and yang, such as acid and alkaline balance. The body attempts self-regulation by eliminating any excess or with malfunction of organs. To avoid such reactions to animal foods, we can balance the yang of animal foods by eating them with potato, salad, or tomato or, in the case of fish, with grated radish. Vinegar sauce, wine, or sugar are often eaten with animal foods for balance. This kind of diet, however, may be allowed in a very cold season or climate, but will bring tragedy such as sickness, war, crime, and violence when it is applied in a warmer climate, tropical, or semitropical zone. Man's tragedies are violations of the Order of the Universe.

B. Vegetarianism

Meat-eating violates the constitution of the Order of Man. Even though meat-eating has advantages such as making man grow faster, fatter, and stronger, it will cause the lose of originality, independence, and biological abnormality. Meat-eating is a biological grafting of the seed of man on animals instead of on vegetables. Meat-eating is an artificially distorted means to becoming a man instead of a natural means. Meat-eating produces an unfree man who acts violently, desires greedily, and thinks egoistically.

Seven times more land is required to raise cattle than to grow vegetables. Therefore, it is a natural result that meat-eating has caused fighting for land (territory) in many forms—diplomatic, economical, cultural, and armed war. If everyone were to eat meat, even though it improves muscle strength, a shortage of land may result. The present social cry for population control is nothing but a result of meat-eating. Population control by pills or other chemicals is based on a mentality of convenience and ego-centered thinking. In the long run, this method will cause a destruction of society and morality.

However, nobody can change one's pleasure. Therefore, I do not push anybody to change his diet to vegetarianism when he likes to eat meat. I am only saying that man's diet is basically vegetables allowing about 10 percent animal foods as a pleasure. In fact, Western vegetarianism is a reaction of Westerners to the recent custom of carnivorism, which produces an acidic condition. This acidic condition has attracted them to vegetables. They are vegetarians because they feel better by eating vegetables only or, because of sentimentality, they do not wish to see animals killed. If animal foods did not cause any trouble, they would eat animal foods. When science scares us by saying that one cannot properly grow without eating 100 grams of meat or eggs everyday, then this sentimental vegetarianism ends. Western vegetarianism lacks principles that ancient Eastern religion has. If the principle of vegetarianism is not understood, lacking any history of vegetarianism, and due to climatic conditions, Western vegetarianism will not last long.

On the other hand, Macrobiotic vegetarianism is not a reaction but is based on thousands of years of religious teachings, cosmology, and their practical application in daily life. Therefore, in order to understand macrobiotics, one must understand the principles of vegetarianism, which I am writing here.

It is a scientific fact that there are more herbivorous animals than carnivorous animals and that the former live longer. In other words, vegetables are more suited to animals than animal foods. Vegetable foods are not only health-giving but also medicinal when they are properly selected, cooked, and eaten.

C. Grains, the Main Foods of Man

Within vegetables, grains are the most important food for men. The reasons for this are as follows:

1. Another name for grain is "cereal," which is derived from Ceres, the Roman goddess of grains and of the harvest. Grains have been cultivated from time immemorial and have been main foods for man except recently in civilized countries.

2. Grains are the most abundant foods on earth and most of the population on earth are living on grains. This is shown on the following statistics.

Grains and Other Productions of Grains, 1970–1971
(Unit in Million Ton)

	USA	World
Wheat	44.6	313.6
Oats	12.7	52.5
Corn	140.7	291.3

Barley	10.1	132.6
Rice (milled)	2.5	195.6
Soybeans	31.8	43.4
Edible vegetables and oils	6.1	20.6
Meat	18.8	

3. The modern nutritional theory recommends eggs and animal protein as the best source of foods or the most important foods. However, I disagree with this from my 40 years of experience in curing sicknesses. Grains, beans, and vegetables may contain fewer amino-acids than animal foods but they are far superior foods for man. As long as medicine believes in animal foods, sicknesses of man will never be cured, and man will never be happy.

4. From the macrobiotic viewpoint, there are many grades of yin and yang in vegetables and grains. I have defined the grade of man as K/Na ± 5-7/1. To this grade, grains are closer to the grade of man than that of vegetables, which are mostly between 20 to 600. Therefore, if one eats vegetables without proper cooking for a long time, one eventually ends up with extreme yin conditions such as introversion, worry, loneliness, exclusivity, alienation, melancholy, supersensitivity, and suspicion. They will suffer from many sicknesses—rheumatism, arthritis, hearing diseases, tuberculosis, epilepsy, polio, miscarriage, ulcer, high blood pressure, cancer, mental sickness (retardation, schizophrenia), etc.

Fruits are more yin (contain more potassium) than vegetables. Therefore, fruits have stronger effects on us. When we eat fruits indiscriminately, they may cause the above sicknesses, while raw vegetables are less likely to do so. Sugar, vinegar, coffee, and spices are generally more yin than fruits. Yin foods, raw vegetables and fruits, can be well balanced foods for those who are extremely yang persons, due to long-time meat-eating. Also, raw vegetables and some local seasonal fruits will be ideal foods in hot weather or locality.

Contrary to the above, excess yang, that is to say when the ratio K/Na is smaller than 4/1, will cause sicknesses. Eating excess yang, one may suffer from the following sicknesses: appendicitis, night walking, dancing sickness, elephantiasis, Addison's disease, liver disease, jaundice, etc.

Right Cooking

So far I have defined what the right foods for man are. The next important thing in the macrobiotic diet is cooking. Why is cooking necessary? Is it necessary at all?

Cooking is the preliminary process of digestion and assimilation of vegetal foods by animals who don't have the ability of autotropism (ability to transmute inorganic matter into organic matter or ability to produce organic matter from inorganic matter). In other words, cooking is a helping technique for the transmutation of vegetables to animals (yin to yang). Practically speaking, cooking is a method to reduce water, potassium (K), vitamin C (all are yin), by fire, pressure, dehydration, and salt, which are all yang, so that yin vegetables are yangized. These yangized vegetables will be digested and assimilated in the mouth, stomach, and intestine and finally changed to animal cells. Because the final products (animal cells) are more yang than the beginning of the process (vegetable cells), this cooking process is yangizing. However, yang foods, like meat, use yin methods instead of yang methods by using sugar, vinegar, or wine to take out the blood.

From this cooking principle, yang vegetables such as jinenjo (mountain potato), carrot, scallion, etc. do not require yang cooking. On the other hand, strong yin foods such as eggplant and potato require good yang methods of fire, dehydration, and salt, etc.

Yin salad is good for the hot (yang) summer or with animal foods. Russian salad is not so yin because their climate is cold (yin). A meat-eater should eat more yin salad than a vegetarian. In the

Western countries, fruits are highly valued. The reason for this is in the fact that they eat lots of meat which is yang. However, an excess of fruits will cause Basedow's disease (exophthalmic goiter), uterus retroflexion, abnormal menstruation, heart disease, falling hair, near-sightedness, astigmatism, detached retina, deafness, miscarriage, frigidity, tuberculosis, cataract, glaucoma, rheumatism, arthritis, polio, hydrocephalus, etc.

The most common yinnizing agent is water. Intake of excess water may cause the yin sicknesses mentioned above. Generally speaking, fruits are 10 times more yin than water because the K/Na of fruits is large (usually 100-1,000:1). Sugar is 20 times more yin than fruits. One tablespoon of sugar is more yin than 10 tangerines. However, vinegar is much more yin than sugar. An excess of chemical vinegar may cause bladder stone, kidney stone, bladder infection, rheumatism, frigidity, arthritis, heart disease, etc.

Living is a yang phenomena. Therefore, excess yin is suicidal. However, animal life must depend on vegetables—yin (read previous chapter). This is the reason that cooking is necessary. Man's civilization started by the invention of salt and fire, and both of them are yang. Ancient man worked for salt. The origin of the word "salary," is salt. The main roads made by the Roman Empire were to serve for the transportation of salt. The main composition of blood is salt. The Japanese word "Chi Shio" literally means "salt of the earth" or "salt on earth," and the normal meaning is blood. Without salt, animals cannot live.

Fermentation by bacteria or enzyme is a yin method of cooking. Miso and tamari, however, are aged for a long time (which is yang), contain lots of salt (which is again yang), and are very yang products even though they are the products of fermentation. Dried bonita is an extremely clever product of fermentation. At first, it is fermented by yin bacteria, and then the yin bacteria is eliminated by dehydration (yang), sunshine, heat (yang), and yang bacteria (penicillium). It is a wonderful thing that this kind of food process was invented more than a thousand years ago.

In short, cooking is an important part of macrobiotic medicine.

One who wants to master macrobiotic medicine must master cooking thoroughly.

Right Eating and Activity

If you eat with bad manners or in a disorderly fashion, you cannot build good health even though you select good foods and cook well. How to eat is another important factor of macrobiotic medicine because eating is a ceremony of the creation of life. Because eating is a ceremony of the creation of life, there is an order in eating, that is to say, order in yin and yang. You must eat from yang foods to yin foods. Any dinner course has this order—an order of main course, vegetables, dessert, and beverage. If you eat dessert first, you will lose your appetite. If you drink a yang drink after a heavy meal, you may vomit. The traditional table manner of Japan is very restrictive on this point. They teach that three times more grains should be eaten than other foods at one meal. By this, one will observe a good proportion of grains and vegetables. Most nonmacrobiotic Americans eat more vegetables than grains according to my observation. When beginning macrobiotics, change the ratio of grains to vegetables gradually. However, as you follow the macrobiotic diet longer, strive to attain the ratio of 3:l (grains:vegetables). Try to eat with other people as often as possible. This will not only make you sociable but also will help you to eat moderately. Share the foods that you like most so that you will not overeat. Most people eat too large an amount of their favorite foods. This is the first step to sickness and an egoistic attitude. If you have a quart of ice cream, share it with other friends so that you can eat only one tablespoonful. If you eat secretly by yourself because you don't want it to be known that you are eating ice cream or if you want to eat by yourself because of your greediness, you will end up with a headache, tiredness, or no energy. This is a social order in eating.

The last important suggestion on eating is chew well and work hard. The Japanese word equivalent to "work" is "hataraku," which literally means to make others relaxed and let them have a good time. If a wife works hard, her husband can have an easy time. If a husband works hard, his wife can have a leisure time. You sleep about one-third of the day because others are working for you. Then you should work for others when you are up. If you don't do this, your life will lack order. Whenever you eat good foods, if you do not work for yourself or others (for example, for your wife and children), the blood that is made by the good foods you eat will not circulate well enough in the body and will cause stagnation. This stagnant blood causes sickness. In other words, eating good foods is not enough to be healthy and happy. You should work hard at least a few hours a day, even those who are sick and have difficulty moving. In fact, this is the secret of the macrobiotic medicine. I say this, because I saw many people who recovered from sickness easily and those people are always good, hard workers. I do not mean working others to the point of slavery. Your work must be your own and original. If you don't have such work, you can do sweeping or cleaning or dish-washing or anything around the house. This work is not for others. This is for your own health and happiness. To those who do not understand this, my medicine is useless.

Summary

I summarize the regular macrobiotic diet, here, for convenience:

1. Biologically speaking, man should eat mainly vegetables.

2. Economically and ecologically speaking, 50 percent or more of foods should be grains. [Editor's note: For the long-time meat-eaters, this high amount of grains will be difficult at first. Therefore, it may be wise to change gradually. Please read *Macrobiotics: An Invitation to Health and Happiness*.]

3. Thirty percent of the diet will be vegetables (nuts, beans, vegetables, and seaweeds).

4. The rest (20 percent) will be any foods including animals and fruits. However, this does not include chemically produced foods or foods with chemical additives.

5. Cooking: Learn to add the best amount of salt, individually. Start the diet with a small amount of salt. Then increase it very slowly until you find the best condition of body and mind.

6. Condiments: Salt and vegetable oil are the most important condiments. Authentically made miso and tamari are very good condiments, especially miso, which is so important that it is a food rather than a condiment. The amount of miso and tamari should be decided upon individually and by the season if you cook by yourself. If you live in another's home, try to adjust this by the amount you eat. In other words, if the foods cooked are too salty, don't eat too much. Eat only foods that fit you. Small fish or seaweed can be used as a condiment (less than 10 percent of total food). Use only a small quantity of spices.

7. Drinking: No alcohol and less coffee.

8. Eating: Eat according to hunger. Chew well—at least 30-100 times each mouthful.

9. Snacks: It is better to have no snacks.

10. Try to eat foods that grow nearest to you. This is the recognition of the law of "Shin Do Fu Ji" (body and soil is one). In other words, body is a transformation of soil. Eating foods that come from far away will cause illness if yin and yang balance is not maintained. If you should eat foods that come from far away, you should be careful to balance yin and yang.

Vegetables growing in colder (yin) climate are yang because such vegetables accumulate more yang elements than yin elements by the law that yin attracts yang. A man who eats such foods becomes yang and can survive and maintain a good balance with the colder climate. However, if he eats vegetables that have grown in a warmer climate, he becomes yin and will not be able to stand a colder climate because the warmer (yang) climate produces yin vegetables, by the same mechanism I mentioned above.

Here, I end the simple explanation of Macrobiotics. In order to cure sickness macrobiotically, you must understand the principle of macrobiotics that I have written here and in other books. Please read and reread them well before you apply my method of macrobiotic treatment for curing sickness.

Part 2

Curing Sickness

Manual of Macrobiotics

From the Ohsawa Lectures
Written by Nina Bond

Macrobiotics is not a mystique. It is the art of life, the simple application of the Unique Principle, Yin and Yang.

But its results, immediate and long-lasting, appear magical...

Self-applied, it diagnoses, prescribes, treats, and cures. Analytical, yet leading to unification, it is an everyday guide to perfect health, absolute justice, infinite freedom, or, in one word, happiness.

It is applicable to everything and everybody, everywhere under the sun.

Without metaphysical or mythological assay, without dogma, without creed, macrobiotics is a self-ordained therapy on a physical and psychological level for those involved and suffering in existence.

Not a bloodless cult, nor an embalmed, dry-as-dust discourse assembled for the benefit of the academy, macrobiotics ignores chatter of the abstract, the impersonal, all intellectual constructs, concepts and systems that do not delineate the salvation of the physical man. "Professors of what another man has suffered," Kierkegaard called the philosophers of the West.

Macrobiotics is for you, here and now, today and forever. But you must be your own doctor. No one can purify or save another. Subjectivity is the measurement of truth.

The macrobiotic discipline is direct, self-reliant, and self-sufficient. It is a do-it-yourself method and process of healing, of change, of transmutation. To become macrobiotic and thus, invulnerable, you have first to will to so become. You alone can exercise your will. Perfection is not a thing acquired from outside, but the realization of the potential within you. And the Unique Principle is the instrument to convert potential into realization.

Will is of prime importance here. Then the word "do." You must do. Action, not intellectualization, leads to knowledge. Think and argue all you like, you will not think a way to heaven. Mere thinking never gained man an inch in stature. Action alone will heal and set you free.

Sooner or later you will find the formulae of the intellect contradictory. Plunge into experience. Enter upon the macrobiotic way. It is the only way you will come to truly know and understand yourself and, it follows, the entire universe. Man is a microcosm of the universe.

The first step is the repair and restoration of the physical self. Nourish your body with the constituent forces of the universe by means of the macrobiotic diet. Systematically rid yourself not only of the gross aspects of disease and discomfort, the biological physicality, but also those disorders of the psyche termed paranoia, egomania, schizophrenia, neuroses, all "mental illness." Characterological changes go along with physical ones.

However, do not undertake the macrobiotic discipline lightly, as a whim, or because you are bored or depressed. Do not undertake it at all unless you are interested in pursuing the principle behind it. Yin/Yang is an ancient and honorable principle, a tried and true way of life. Trifle with it to your sorrow.

Be warned!

If you decide to embark upon the macrobiotic way, know that you will change. Your whole life will change. It is inescapable, unavoidable. Nor is such change as one writ upon the waters. Deepgraven, it will remain impressed on the very foundation of your existence. And, once having experienced the effects of the Unique Principle, you will not be able to forget it no matter how hard you try. It is ineradicable. For the Unique Principle is harmony, and its memory never sleeps.

After a period, when you have nourished body and mind the macrobiotic way, remembering proportion, and combining in yourself the bitter, the pungent, the salt, and the sweet, balancing your food intake between Yin and Yang, it may occur to you for some reason, or for none at all, to forsake the Unique Principle, to forget the whole thing.

Understand before you begin that you will not be allowed to forget. Not only will your body protest and memory haunt the hours of your day, but the inner man, your own true self, having tasted the elusive nectar, having ventured, even briefly, over the border into the long yearned-for state called harmony, called happiness, called peace, called grace, will evermore plague you seeking return.

If you are perfectly happy now, content with your life and free of doubt about the future, there is no need for you to experiment with Yin and Yang. But if after sober consideration, you make up your mind to embrace the Unique Principle and undertake the macrobiotic way, then observe closely, *in toto*, your present condition; note carefully the factors you wish to change, to be rid of, to heal, or to destroy, and which elements you want transmuted into others.

The macrobiotic discipline is nothing if not revolutionary. Exercising it, you will completely remake and remold your character, your body, and your brain.

Is it a physical ailment, a bodily complaint, you wish to cure? Or one of the mind (mind in its comprehensive sense of heart, intellect, and affection; and in the philosophical sense as subject, substance, or soul)? You can tap and activate, or reactivate, dormant and long-hidden resources, physical and psychic, with macrobiotics.

This means, also, that you will reactivate old sores, old wounds and bruises. Forgotten abscesses, concealed cankers deep-buried in body and consciousness, are brought to the surface, brought out into the light, where they fade and pass away, heated at last, and forgotten.

First, re-establish communication with your body. It speaks to you quite clearly. Learn to read its messages accurately.

If you are suddenly seized with a cramp in the leg or foot (the most Yang parts of the body), think back. What have you been eating? Was it the acid (Yin) of fruit or berries? The chemicals and sugar (both extreme Yin) of a carbonated beverage?

Are you frequently angry? Apprehensive, or even terrified, for no apparent reason? Fear is Yin. Introduce fear's Yang counterpart into your diet. Yangize yourself. Fear is nullified if Yang courage and strength are added.

Do people conspire against you, try to get your job, your money, your wife? Are you a heavy meat-eater (Yang)?

Is your husband sadistic, cruel, sexually demanding? Learn the foods that tame; prepare and serve them to him.

Are you, a man, too passive and feminine (Yin)? And is your wife strident, assertive, domineering? She is too Yang. Change yourselves; assume your proper role and character in the drama of life. Realize your true nature by eating in accord with the Unique Principle. Balance Yin with Yang.

Were you a sickly, frightened child? Did you suffer some trauma that hindered the natural development of your young man or womanhood? The remnants of that illness or injury will manifest itself during the macrobiotic discipline for a brief moment, to be viewed, endured, and understood by you, then dissolve and disappear forever.

With the macrobiotic diet, you can erase all past mistakes, rectify all error. You can become clean and pure, as in the beginning, the jewel of your essence shining with its original brilliance. You can become as the Uncarved Block (wood as it comes from the tree), Raw Silk (before it is printed or dyed), or the Newborn Child (natural and simple and good, before social influences prevail upon it).

Any physical disorder; the useless burden of anxiety, vague or defined; the myriad confusions of purpose, of ideals, of thoughts, and attitudes; feelings of guilt for acts of omission or commission; all, but all, can be transmuted into their opposites simply by employing the compass of Yin and Yang, and the energy that supported unnatural disorder, anxiety, confusion, and guilt, is released for its own pure and natural intended use.

You have become you, clean and new, invulnerable before the host and multitude of poisons (social and chemical), the flood-tide of Western civilization forces upon a for-the-most-part unsuspecting world. You are macrobiotic. You are free!

The macrobiotic man or woman walks in total freedom, completely healthy and happy in body, the mind a shining arrow that penetrates stone or star with equal ease. The Ideal Man. A living, breathing demonstration of the timeless, immutable law of changes.

So combine in yourself the bitter, the pungent, the salt, and the sweet—in proportion. Balance Yin and Yang. Then, in wholehearted accord with all of life, in close harmony with what is past, passing, and yet to come, proceed along your way.

Everything you see and do and are stands revealed to you, each in its own clear essence and meaning. Colors are brighter, truer, deeper. Heat and cold remain what they have always been but you experience them for what they are: heat and cold, no more, no less. Your breath is ever sweet, your heart is light, your step is joyous.

You are macrobiotic and nothing is impossible to you!

Preparation

You are superior to other animals, and you must cure yourself at least as simply as they do (birds, fish, insects, even bacteria). If you are unable to realize your own infinite freedom, eternal happiness, and absolute integrity [droiture (French): must be understood as both honesty and wholeness as well as justice], then you deserve to harbor worms, viruses, and destructive bacteria in your body and don't have to fear hell after death because you are living it now. [Consider today's degenerative diseases, neuroses, guilt, paranoia, malaise; fear of atomic holocaust, overpopulation, fear of the future, boredom.]

Caring for your health is the most significant spiritual thing you can do. If more primitive forms of life stay healthy without medicines, doctors, and hospitals, why not you too?

Every man should be happy. If you aren't, then you personally are a criminal sentenced to slavery by the Order of the Universe. If you choose to serve the sentence, then your supreme judgment was or still is partly or completely blocked. If you choose to be happy (free, independent, in good health, joyous, friend to everyone everywhere, always) and to live a long life, you must first restore your intuition (your innate supreme judgment) by following the correct way of eating, in harmony with nature geographically and seasonally, as revealed with deep understanding by the ancient Chinese and Indian philosophies (in the *Nei-King*, the *I-King*, the *Charak Samhita,* and the *Gitas)*, the basis of the oldest and highest civilizations known to us.

Man is born free, healthy, sane, welcome in all men's eyes, without artifice, without weapons; he is born in harmony with the Order of the Universe.

We can remain in this state if we choose to. Why not?

Nothing is easier than treating disease and unhappiness. After all, treating disease is just rejecting the use of traumatic, gory violence in our everyday life and eating. It means returning ourselves to the Order of the Universe and to our Infinite Self.

Nothing is easier than regaining paradise—everybody knows the key—the cross, the Star of David, the double fish symbol of Yin and Yang. In Japan, newborn babies have embroidered on their first clothes the Star of David.

Infinite freedom, eternal happiness, and absolute integrity are not hard to come by—what else is there is our spiritual world? From all time we are given everything.

Overcoming unhappiness even in this finite relative world is simple—there are no lasting oppressors or enslaving rules. Besides, the relative world is just a point in the space of the infinite universe.

Nothing is easier or greater fun than dealing with this world's troubles because we can view them for what they are: The interplay of yin and yang. Life is really wonderful when we hold this yin/yang compass as our guide!

Let lawyers, businessmen, policemen, professors, all usurers, and slave-makers be damned!

1. First, you must persevere in the most direct, least expensive path toward eternal happiness, infinite freedom, and absolute integrity. No need for money or gear for this new trip. As Jesus told his disciples before a long journey into unknown countries: "Take only one undergarment and no baggage." The only preparation is psychological. Follow the way of eating and soon you will understand, fully, Epictetus when he said: "If you are not happy, it is your own fault."

This means you are born happy, free, full of love and justice. If you are not happy and free, if you are sick and dependent on others, then you are ignoring nature's laws, the Order of the Universe that you knew even before your birth without ever learning it. So-called education blinds you to this order. Justice demands that you suffer whether you be victim or accomplice, just as a certain dose of poison will kill you whether you take it wittingly or unwittingly.

The duration of your unhappiness depends on the length and number of your crimes. You may break society's laws because they change with every generation; lawmakers are sometimes hung. But beware lest you ignore the Order of Man. Ignorance of the law is never an attenuating circumstance. If your prison cell is sickness or unhappiness, then you are serving a sentence dealt out by the Order of Man. You can get around society's laws with money, bribery, fraud, violence, or revolution. There's no escaping natural law; it is so perfect. It is all-inclusive. [The Order of the Universe is the justice of yin and yang constantly and dynamically interacting. It encompasses the whole relative world. We cannot break this order (law); we cannot get outside it.] The only way is to change your own thinking and your own view of life to harmonize with this universal order. If you do not accept Epictetus' words, it is useless for you to read on. You can save your time.

2. Only man, of all the animals, has changed this world into one of madness, unhappiness, sickness, crime, murder, and warfare. Look at birds, rats, mosquitoes, butterflies, wolves. They really enjoy life; they are truly satisfied, happy, and peaceful. You never saw a tiger with a headache, a toothache, indigestion, or rheumatism; a crow buying aspirin; an old buck wearing glasses; a cow with gonorrhea; a calf dying of measles. You never saw a lion bloated like a domestically raised pig. If man is really the most highly-developed animal, then he should be free of all sickness. No pack of wolves wage war on another; they don't torture and slaughter each other. Man is always fighting man. Indeed, we have made ourselves lower than any other animal. We must understand how this came about.

3. Only man depends on other people and on artificial means for his health and happiness. Animals cure themselves and help each other. Why cannot man do likewise?

4. Once you are cured, participate in our world health program; go out and visit people paralyzed with disease; tell them what you

have done, how you have healed yourself; give, or sell, as many of these books as possible. You should be able to heal at least a hundred people. This is not a purely altruistic act; it trains you as a macrobiotic artist. Many new problems will challenge you. Write back and ask us for advice. All this time you will be sharpening your judgment and widening your knowledge of the macrobiotic way of eating. You will begin to appreciate the real nature of health and life based on freedom and happiness. And you will become a happy man within your society.

If you can heal an average of 30 people in three months and inspire them to do the same, there will soon be hundreds and thousands of macrobiotic healers in this country.

You will be helping doctors, nurses, the minister of health, and the United Nations. To convince people who have been suffering uselessly for years on end, just get them committed to trying your "primitive" and inexpensive way of eating. It's not hard. Tell them of your own experience, our simple practical suggestions, and you'll be finished in an hour. An hour a day is not too much to sacrifice. Really, it is no sacrifice because you will become more accomplished in the art of healing and, at the same time, surer in your self-healing. If you cannot spare this hour a day, you will become unhappy again very soon no matter what you do after your "cure;" one of your children, your wife, husband, or family, maybe you yourself will suffer from the same or a new disease. (In the first instance, the same cure will not work, and I personally make a practice of never treating the same person for the same sickness twice!).

If you are unable to discover the cure for all your family's, your town's, and your society's sicknesses, then quite soon you will become more and more exclusive, self-centered, arrogant, and lonesome. Your unhappiness is relative to the number of friends you have and your ability to make new ones. A free man appreciates all other men; he is at home everywhere and is open to everything.

5. Make a personal evaluation at the end of each week using the seven conditions of health. If you don't make some progress each week and a great improvement after two months, you are doing

something wrong. Stop your self-healing; either you are too careless or not really committed to leading a free and happy life.

6. Always stay in touch with some macrobiotic center. Send questions, personal progress reports, and word of your social activities so the center can send you its publications, news, and suggestions. (For information about the center closest to you or for more information on macrobiotics, contact the George Ohsawa Macrobiotic Foundation at *www.ohsawamacrobiotics.com*.)

Preliminary Suggestions

Here is the kind of prescription I give to a sick person seeking health: Dear friend, If you are really committed to curing all man's sicknesses and your own, if modern medicine has given you up as "hopeless," if you have been suffering for a long time and long to reach heaven, infinite freedom, eternal happiness, and absolute integrity as soon as possible, please follow these steps very conscientiously.

Here is the soundest advice I can give you after 40 years of treating "hopeless" cases in Japan. Send me a daily progress report telling me:

1. your psychological state (happy or not, relaxed or tense).

2. the quantity and quality of food and drink you consume.

3. the regularity and changes of your bowel movements and urinations.

Without this daily report, I am unable to work out the way to change your physical condition.

Preliminary Diet

(Do not stay on this diet more than one month without consulting a more experienced person.)

1. Drink only the amount of liquid necessary to maintain your health. Take into account water, tea, soup, and liquid in food.

2. Exclude all sugar, spices, chilies, curries, pepper, vinegar, alcohol, and animal products. [The original diet also excluded potatoes, tomatoes, and eggplant as well as fruit and did not include alcohol among the taboo items; but, present thinking is that some

fruit, in season and local, as well as properly prepared potatoes, to-matoes, and eggplant help discharge meat toxins, which are so heavy in Americans and Westerners beginning macrobiotics. The yin effect of alcohol is more deleterious in that it passes directly into the blood stream and does not pass through the digestive system's neutralizing course as do these solid foods. Occasionally, fish may in some cases be recommended. See *Chico-San Cookbook; Do of Cooking, Vol. 1-4*; *Macrobiotics: An Invitation to Health and Happiness; Cooking with Grains and Vegetables;* and *Cooking Good Food,* pages 2-4.]

3. Eat the following: whole brown rice, wheat, buckwheat, rolled or whole oats, barley, millet, corn or cornmeal, all unrefined. Do not throw away cooking water. Prepare them by frying, toasting, soaking, sautéing; then boiling, baking, pressure cooking. Eat small amounts of vegetables (leaves, roots, tubers) like cabbage, cauliflower, onion, carrot, pumpkin, radish, dandelion, cress, endive, salsify, celery, es-pecially cooked without water or sautéed and seasoned with sea salt. They should be locally grown, within a 500-mile radius, and native to the country. Use only unrefined sesame or corn oil.

4. Proportions: grains 70-90 percent, and vegetables 10-30 per-cent is best. [Ohsawa was not directing this to post-psychedelic America and, so, some of his recommendations should, we feel, be tempered. Eating a broader spectrum and less fanatic salt intake seems advisable in 2010, USA. Please see *Rice and the Ten Day Rice Diet; Macrobiotics: An Invitation to Health and Happiness;* and *Do of Cooking, Vol. 1.*]

5. Chew thoroughly. At least 50 times. More is better. The longer you chew each mouthful, the faster you will be cured.

6. It is very important to be constantly adjusting your daily in-take to the minimum necessary. Any superfluousness, either in quan-tity or quality, reduces your happiness. Waste, luxury, and plain indulgence all lead to crime and slavery: unhappiness, depression, sickness, poverty, indecision, mediocre suffering, premature-death by disease or accident, continuing slavery.

Through this diet you will discover the daily waste you have been committing. The complete freedom, unlimited happiness and joy, the wholeness you will experience come simply from eating according to the unifying principle of yin and yang, in small amounts.

Since food is the *sine qua non* of our life and our activity, overeating or wasting that which may be of use to others is nothing less than killing by negligence. This, then, is the basics that leads to sound memory and thinking, the natural social good sense and intuition that modern education has repressed in us.

All man's unhappiness, even war, is the result of bad judgment. Self-indulgence, sentimental thinking, "scientific" theorizing typical in Western analysis, all lead to greed, intolerance, and inability to see the whole (this is Supreme Judgment), and blind us to the light and the works that were the core of all the great Eastern religions.

This way of healing is a practical simplified version of the yogic and Buddhist way of eating, the first step to self-realization and freedom from enslavement and immediate sensory gratification—Gandhi's ideal and that of his guru Rajchandra.

Self-realization opens us to our own innate Supreme Judgment, which is itself infinite freedom, eternal happiness, and absolute integrity. Becoming whole and invulnerable to the fracturing forces of our world is everyone's goal, but few really pursue it in their daily lives. Life is a dynamic swing between the perfect and the imperfect. Man still doesn't know where and how to find the path, yet it is so easy and so enjoyable, the *only* way to eternal happiness.

Remember, I cannot cure the same person of the same sickness twice because my way is the way of continuing healing always leading to health, peace, and freedom.

Special Diet

Quick cure: If you are committed to curing yourself by yourself, as soon as possible, despite temporary apparent regressions, you should follow this diet at least two months.

1. Complete fasting one or two days or weeks (no food, but with liquids) or continue with less liquid and your usual work pace.

2. Omit completely all sugar, spices, chilies, curries, pepper, vinegar, alcohol, fruit, and animal products, including dairy. Later,

when you have reached a level of relative good health and you feel an irresistible craving, you may take small amounts of these things (except, of course, sugar).

3. Proportion of grains to vegetables 60 percent grains to 40 percent vegetables for yang persons; 85 percent grains to 15 percent vegetables for yin persons—by weight before cooking.

4. Stop all chemical drugs and other therapies.

5. Keep as physically active as possible.

Keep a diary of what you eat and drink, in what combinations, and of your psychological changes.

After hearing these don'ts, people often ask, "So what can we eat...?" These people are simple-headed, self-centered gourmands. And that is why they are sick and unhappy. They are unwittingly confessing their selfishness, their original sin—which they are still committing unknowingly—of bad eating. Their judgment cannot proceed beyond the third level.

They are ignorant of the hundreds of different plants in the world and of the thousands of ways of preparing them, which any good cook knows. Tokyo's best restaurant is Tokyo Kaikan, with several large dining halls and hundreds of smaller dining rooms. There they serve French, Italian, English, Chinese, and Japanese dishes— even the famous bouillabaisse of Prunier. The main chef there, Mr. Tanaka, stated publicly that he is entirely convinced of the culinary and physiological superiority of the macrobiotic way of eating. "At Tokyo Kaikan, we know how to prepare any dish for our customers but I myself prefer my wife's cooking according to Mr. Ohsawa's teaching"

The art of cooking is the art of creating life. Our health and our resulting happiness, freedom, and thinking ability depend on it. That is why in the great Buddhist centers and orthodox monasteries only the highest disciples may become cooks.

Cooking is the basis of all man's spiritual and physical development. If only Professor Herrigel, author of *Japanese Archery*, had studied this oldest of Japanese arts! Why did he die so young? Because he was looking for technical perfection without the philosophy behind it.

The highest dreams of man: happiness and health, freedom and peace, must have a firm foundation in biology, physiology, and dialectics. Otherwise, they can never be fulfilled. Despite lesser faults and centuries of hardships, a nation cultured in the unifying principle of yin and yang and in its basic biological, physiological, and dialectic application will endure.

If you don't cook already, study. Be creative—be a creator. Otherwise, you remain a slave to life's vicissitudes.

If your patient doesn't appreciate your cooking, if he has no appetite and refuses to eat, don't worry. All sick men overeat, consciously or unconsciously. They should be eating less or even fasting, as Jesus, Buddha, and other great spiritual leaders practiced and taught.

Macrobiotic Internal Treatment

(For further details, refer to chapter "Cooking for the Sick")

Bancha Twig Tea: Helps purify your blood and is good for fatigue, weakness, heart conditions, gonorrhea, syphilis, nephritis; daily use. (See recipe 65.)

Chrysanthemum Tea: This is a light drink for daily use. Very good for children once a month. Excellent for intestinal worms, especially round worms. Good for weakness. (See recipe 53.)

Mugwort Tea (yomogi or armoise): Good as a daily drink and for worms. Strengthens the heart and stomach. (See recipe 47.)

Tamari Bancha (syoban): For extreme fatigue or weakness. Its effect is strengthening and refreshing. Good for heart conditions, rheumatism, stomach aches, especially heartburn, ulcers, and indigestion. (See recipe 43.)

Umesho Bancha (salt plum tea): Same as Tamari Bancha but stronger. Especially good for anemia. Promotes good blood circulation. (See recipe 44.)

Brown Rice Soup: This is good for all sicknesses. (See recipe 54.)

Brown Rice Tea: Good for all sicknesses or as a daily summer drink. (See recipe 41.)

Gomasio (sesame salt): Good for all sicknesses. Used daily, it strengthens the body's resistance by setting up a good intracellular potassium/extracellular sodium ratio. (See recipe 67.)

Rice Coffee: Especially recommended for students and others doing intellectual work. Helps clarify ideas. Good for constipation and recurring headaches. (See recipe 55.)

Miso (fermented soybean puree): For heart conditions, diabetes, rheumatism, polio, asthma, and especially tuberculosis. Helpful to smokers as it will eliminate nicotine from the blood stream. Used for healthy skin. (See recipes 20, 48, 49, 50.)

Yannoh (grain drink): Made from roasted grains, beans and roots. Yangizes and revitalizes. (See recipe 68.)

Kokkoh (grain milk): Made from roasted whole brown rice or half-and-half brown and sweet rice, wheat berries, brown sesame seeds and soybeans. Grind to a fine powder and use as powdered milk to substitute for mother's milk. (See recipe 56 and *Milk, A Myth of Civilization.*)

Kuzu (Japanese arrowroot): Soothing and stimulating. Extremely good for sharp intestinal pains, diarrhea, dysentery, cholera, and intestinal tuberculosis. (See recipe 57.)

Umesho Kuzu: Same as Umesho Bancha, and especially good for diarrhea. (See recipe 58.)

Thick Buckwheat Cream (soba flour): Necessary to build strong constitutions. Fine for all cancers, kidney and lung diseases, especially kidney tuberculosis. (See recipe 9.)

Bajra (a variety of millet grown at altitudes of 300 feet or more in a cold dry climate; "Hie" in Japanese): Used for strengthening the body, especially in cold weather. (See recipe 59.)

Shio Kombu: Very effective in curing arterial diseases, varicose veins, goiter, hemorrhoids, and especially arteriosclerosis. (See recipe 60.)

Mochi (sweet rice cakes): Good for nursing mothers with lack of milk. Very effective for eliminating all kinds of stones from the body and for building flexible muscles. (See recipes 2, 5, 61, and *Do of Cooking, Vol. 4,* p. 23.)

Special Rice Soup: Very effective for rheumatism, arthritis, and heart conditions. (See recipe 62.)

Aduki Bean Soup: Very effective for nephritis and diabetes. Good for kidneys. (See recipe 63.)

Daikon Tea No. 1: Fine for fever and chills. Don't use too often. Keep warm after drinking so you perspire and urinate. (See recipe 45.)

Daikon Tea No. 2: Take once a day when stomach is empty, but not more than three days. Good for swelling of legs or feet. This also works for kidney and urination troubles. (See recipe 46.)

Lotus Root Tea: Take one drink three times a day and no other liquid. For asthma, whooping cough, and all other lung diseases. If a baby has whooping cough, the mother is given the tea during the breastfeeding period, but it is never given to the baby. (See recipe 64.)

Raw Brown Rice: A handful of raw rice well-chewed each morning on an empty stomach, for about one month, will rid the duodenum of hookworms.

Rice Cream: Very good for extreme weakness or loss of appetite. (See recipe 11.)

Tekka No. 1: Good for rheumatism, arthritis, and also skin diseases. (See recipe 14.)

Tekka No. 2: Good for coughs and whooping cough. (See recipe 15.)

Tekka No. 3: Good for chest diseases, adenoids, bronchitis, and weak chest. (See recipe 16.)

Macrobiotic External Treatment

(For further details refer to chapter "Procedures for External Treatment")

Ginger compress: Especially recommended for kidney diseases, rheumatism, congestion, convulsions, stomach aches. A ginger hip bath is good for diarrhea. (See recipe 69.)

Albi Plaster (sato-imo in Japan, yucca in America, taro in Africa): Very effective for tuberculosis, appendicitis, pleurisy, rheumatism, arthritis, tumors, skin diseases, including cancer and leprosy. (See recipe 70.)

Tofu Plaster (soybean plaster): This preparation reduces fever rapidly, not physically like ice but pharmaceutically. Never use on chicken pox or measles. (See recipe 71.)

Sesame Oil and Ginger: Good for all headaches, dandruff, and loss of hair. Relieves middle ear inflammation. Very good for rheumatism, skin diseases, and crooked backbone; applied with Ginger Compress. (See recipe 76.)

Sesame Oil: Protects the hair and is effective against grey hair, red hair, and even baldness. Never use mineral oils or any animal-fat-based soaps. (See recipe 74.)

Hibayu (chlorophyll hip bath): Good for skin diseases, bladder inflammation, bed-wetting, menstrual cramps, or other female complaints. (See recipe 75.)

Apple Juice: Relieves headaches when there is no fever. (See recipe 77.)

Radish Juice: Relieves headaches accompanied by fever. (See recipe 78.)

Salt Compress: Calms abdominal pain and diarrhea. (See recipe 79.)

Dentie: Use as a tooth powder. It is the best remedy for pyorrhea and child's toothache. (See recipe 80.)

Nukayu (rice bran): Excellent for eczema. (See recipe 81.)

Carp Plaster: Reduces fever. Effective for pneumonia to break up congestion. (See recipe 72.)

Chlorophyll Plaster (green plaster): Good for fever. Use in place of Albi Plaster when albi is not available. (See recipe 82.)

Hot Foot Bath: Good for blood circulation, kidneys, and insomnia. (See recipe 83.)

Soba Plaster: Especially effective for conditions of bladder and surrounding areas. (See recipe 73.)

Cooking for the Sick
By Lima Ohsawa
Translated by Cornellia Aihara

The following recipes have been applied to sick people in Japan by Mr. Ohsawa and his disciples. In a drug store, the pharmacist prepares drugs designed to cure illness. However, our drug store is a kitchen and the drugs are foods—some of which may be growing in your back yard. You are the pharmacist! Your cooking is the medicine!

Most illnesses are improved in a few months if you follow the preliminary diet. If whoever you are caring for is not improved in several months, you are making some important mistakes in your cooking and/or in the selection of foods. You may need to consult someone who knows macrobiotics better than you.

Months, or even within a few days after starting macrobiotics, it is possible to have a variety of reactions: fever, diarrhea, amenorrhea, cramps, shortness of breath, etc. Do not be alarmed at these reactions—they are the sign of the sick body attempting to reconstruct health—they are nature's operation!

To cure sickness by the macrobiotic diet, you must study macrobiotic principles. Read: *Macrobiotics: An Invitation to Health and Happiness, Seven Basic Macrobiotic Principles, Unique Principle*, and other publications available from the George Ohsawa Macrobiotic Foundation and other publishers to develop your knowledge and understanding of macrobiotics.

Basic rules for cooking are the same as mentioned in the beginning of *Do of Cooking*.

The main foods are:
  A. Whole grains
  B. Preferably cooked with a bit of salt
  C. Organically grown if possible
Secondary foods are:
  a. Local, seasonal vegetables
  b. One-third the amount of main foods (whole grains) is preferable
  c. Avoid foods grown with chemical fertilizers, that have been sprayed, hot-house produced, chemically bleached, or chemically colored
  d. Use the whole food, including the skin wherever possible
  e. Avoid artificial seasonings and condiments
  f. Save cooking juices and stocks to use in cooking
  g. Vegetables should be cooked well except in very yang sickness or for yang persons. Cooking is extremely important for the sick. Well-cooked foods improve appetite, digestion, and assimilation.

Remember, those who are sick and who have observed these macrobiotic principles should consult with someone who has more experience in macrobiotics, especially when reactions continue too long or when there is little or no improvement in their condition for a long time.

Other Information:
  Handful: Always means the amount the patient can hold in one hand.
  Water: For drinking and cooking, should ideally come from a deep well.
  Salt: Is always unrefined white sea salt.
  Sesame Seeds: Should be unhulled. When buying black seeds, be careful to get undyed ones.
  Dyes: Should be scrupulously avoided in all foods as well as artificial coloring.

Recipes

1. Fried Rice Balls (Musubi)

Heat oil in a frying pan. Ease musubi into the hot oil. Fry on each side until a golden brown color. Musubi can also be shaped into flat triangles. Cold musubi fries best. Preheat oil to approximately 350 degrees. If oil is not hot enough, rice balls will taste oily and musubi will absorb too much oil.

2. Mochi Ojiya (soft rice)

4 cups cooked rice	1 cup wild greens (or greens of choice)
5, 2½" square pieces	2 tsp oil
brown rice mochi	Pinch of salt

Deep-fry the brown rice mochi. Cut wild greens (or greens of choice) into small pieces and sauté. Add rice. Add water to cover rice 1-2 inches. Boil about 1 hour until soft and add salt and fried mochi. Cook 20 minutes more. Season with miso, or salt and tamari. Serve with toasted green nori (seaweed). Very good!

3. Millet Kayu (soft cooked)

3⅓ cups millet	12 cups water
1 tsp salt	

Wash millet and add water and salt. Bring to a boil on a high flame and then turn to a low flame, about 20 minutes or until tender.

4. Aduki Millet Kayu

2⅔ cups millet	⅔ cup aduki beans
1 tsp salt	

Cook aduki beans and mix with washed millet. Cook as in recipe 3.

5. Agé-Mochi (fried mochi)

1 lb brown rice mochi	Oil
1½" white daikon	1 Tbsp soy sauce
(radish) grated	

Heat oil in frying pan. Add mochi and fry until both sides are golden brown. Mix daikon and soy sauce. Use as a dip for the mochi. Mochi added to miso soup is good for the weak and for nursing mothers. Can be used everyday.

6. Buckwheat Cream

1⅓ cups buckwheat flour	5 cups water
1 Tbsp oil	Pinch of salt

Heat oil and add buckwheat flour. Sauté a few minutes until roasted. Cool, then add water and bring to a boil. Cook 20 minutes. Add salt. Serve with minced parsley or scallion.

7. Soba Noodle Soup

2¼ cups buckwheat flour	2" carrot
1 cup whole wheat pastry flour	1 bunch scallions
⅔-1⅓ cups cold water	¼ cup wild greens
8 cups water	2 Tbsp oil
1 tsp salt	

Mix buckwheat flour, whole wheat flour, salt, and 1 tablespoon oil with cold water. Knead very well. Roll out very thinly and cut into thin long strips. Cut carrot and wild greens. Sauté in oil. Add 8 cups of water and bring to a boil. Cook until tender. Put soba noodles in the sauce. Bring to a boil. Add salt and soy sauce. Serve with chopped scallion greens or Nori (seaweed).

8. Fried Soba Noodles

1¼ cups buckwheat flour	¼ cup wild greens (or
¾ cup whole wheat flour	greens of choice)
⅔ cup cold water	1 tsp kuzu arrowroot
½ bunch scallions	Pinch of salt
2" carrot	3 Tbsp oil

Mix buckwheat flour, whole wheat flour, and add a pinch of salt. Mix in ⅔ cup of cold water. Knead very well. Roll out very thinly and cut into long thin strips. Add hot water and boil noodles. Drain and fry in 2 tablespoons oil. Sprinkle fried noodles with salt. Serve with vegetable sauce: Cut all vegetables thinly and sauté in 1 tablespoon oil. Add salt, 1⅓ cups cooked noodle water, and bring to a boil. Cook until tender. Season with soy sauce. Mix kuzu with a little cold water and add. Cook for a few minutes, or until thickened and kuzu becomes transparent. Serve fried noodles covered with sauce.

9. Thick Buckwheat Cream

⅔ cup buckwheat flour   Scallions
1 cup boiling water   ¼-½ tsp salt
Soy sauce

Roast buckwheat flour a few minutes in a frying pan, with or without oil. Add boiling water and salt and stir vigorously. Simmer 15-20 minutes until water is absorbed. Let stand 10 more minutes. Sprinkle with chopped scallions, mix with soy sauce, and serve immediately.

10. Sarrasin

(A) Sarrasin with Whole Wheat   (B) Plain Sarrasin
5⅓ cups buckwheat flour   1 cup buckwheat flour
1⅓ cups whole wheat flour   1 Tbsp oil
2 Tbsp oil   ½ tsp salt
2 tsp salt   ½ cup water
3 Tbsp sesame seeds (goma)
2½ cups water

Mix dry ingredients and oil. Add water. Mix well. Bake at 300 degrees for 30-40 minutes.

11. Special Rice Cream

1 cup rice
10 cups water
Pinch of salt

Wash rice. Drain and roast in a dry pan. Stir constantly until golden brown. Add water and bring to a boil. Cook 3-4 hours over low heat, until water is reduced to half. Make a triangle-shaped cotton cloth. With your fingers, press the rice through this cloth bag. You should press out 3–3⅔ cups of rice cream. The bran can be used in breads and muffins. Add a pinch of salt to the rice cream and serve hot. Chew well, the same as other cooked rice.

12. Rice Potage

Cook rice as in recipe 11. Add 3 cups of water to make a thinner mixture.

13. Fried Rice Cream

1 cup rice	Pinch of salt
1 tsp oil	10 cups water

Roast rice in oil and thencook thick as in recipe 11.

14. Tekka No. 1

1 med stalk burdock root	5 dried fish (niboshi) minced,
1½" lotus root	(optional)
½ carrot	1½ cups hacho (mame) miso
1 tsp ginger	(don't use kome (rice) miso!)
⅔ cup sesame oil	

Mince all vegetables very finely, separately. Heat oil in a Chinese frying pan (wok). Sauté burdock until bitter smell is gone. Add niboshi, lotus root, and carrot, in this order. Add ginger and sauté well. Add miso. Mix very well with vegetables. Sauté and cook 3-4 hours over low flame. Cooking it over a low flame is very important. A high flame will not pass through to the inside. Each vegetable must be reached. If cooking with mugi miso, sauté vegetables in ⅓ cup oil first. Then add ⅓ cup of oil before adding miso; continue cooking until moisture is nearly gone. Stir frequently. Consistency should be slightly moist and crumbly when cooled. Serve as a condiment on grains.

15. Tekka No. 2

½ med stalk burdock root	7 niboshi (iriko) (optional)
2" lotus root	1½ cups mame miso
½ stalk carrot	(hacho miso)
1 tsp ginger	⅔ cup sesame oil

Cook as in recipe 14.

16. Tekka No. 3

1 med stalk burdock root	5 niboshi (optional)
3½" lotus root	1½ cups mame miso
½ stalk carrot	⅔ cup sesame oil
1 tsp ginger	

Cook as in recipe 14.

17. Kinpira No. 1

1½ med stalk burdock root, cut sengiri	1 carrot, cut sengiri
2" lotus root, cut sengiri	2 Tbsp oil

Heat oil. Add burdock, sauté well until smell is gone. Add lotus root, carrot, and sauté in that order. Add a bit of water. Cook at medium flame 1 hour with a cover. Add salt and soy sauce. Cook 1 hour more. Take off cover and let all juices mix by shaking and evaporating all moisture.

18. Kinpira No. 2

1 med stalk burdock root	1 carrot
4" lotus root	1 Tbsp oil

Cook as in recipe 17.

19. Kinpira No. 3

½ med stalk burdock root	½ carrot
8" lotus root	1 tsp oil

Cook as in recipe 17.

20. Miso Soup

½ cup wild greens (or greens of choice), cut small	Variation:
⅓ bunch scallion cut ¼"	wakame, daikon, carrots,
4 cups boiling water	burdock, dried daikon,
1 tsp oil	using seasonal vegetables,
⅓ cup mugi miso	two different kinds of
	vegetables

Sauté wild greens. Add scallions, one at a time. Add boiling water. Cook 20-30 minutes or until tender. Add a little boiling water to the mugi miso. Stir well and add to soup. Let come to a boil. Serve immediately. Do not serve more than 2 teaspoons of wild vegetables per person. This is one of the best sources of protein. May be eaten once or twice a day. Can be used as a sauce in place of butter when cooking vegetables.

21. Squash with Aduki Beans

1 cup aduki beans	2 cups squash cut ¾" squares
2" squares kombu	2 cups water

Soak aduki beans 5 hours. Cook beans and kombu with soaked water. Bring to a boil and add ½ cup cold water—repeat two to three times. When they are soft, add the squash. Cook until tender. Season with salt and serve.

22. Hiziki with Lotus Root

2 cups hiziki	2 Tbsp oil
4" lotus root	1-2 Tbsp soy sauce

Wash hiziki, discard washing water, add more water, and soak in cold water for 5 minutes (cover hiziki completely with water). Strain and reserve soaking water. Cut into 1½-inch lengths. Sauté lotus root. Add hiziki and a bit of water (use reserved water). Bring to a boil, add soaking water as necessary, and cook until tender. Season with soy sauce.

23. Waterless-cooked Vegetables

4 cups daikon	4 cups onions
2 cups carrots	

Sauté onions, then daikon and carrots. Yin to yang. Cook, tightly covered, over a low flame until tender. Season with salt and soy sauce. If vegetables start to scorch, use flame-tamer under pot. 1-2 heaping teaspoons per person is recommended serving.

24. Onions and String Beans

To 2 parts onions use 1 part string beans; may cut string beans or cook them whole. Sauté onions, cook until transparent, and add string beans and cook until they change color. Add salt and soy sauce. Cook covered over low flame until tender. Remove cover and shake pan until all juice is mixed with the vegetables, then turn on high flame for just a minute or two.

25. Nira (wild scallions)

Cut nira ½-inch lengths and sauté well in oil. Season with miso. This is a very yang dish.

26. Kiri Boshi Daikon (dried radish)

2 cups dried daikon (soaked in water 20-30 min.)	4 cups water
1 tsp salt	1 Tbsp oil
2 agé, cut thin	1 tsp soy sauce

Cut daikon into ½-inch pieces. Sauté well and add water that daikon soaked in. Add agé and bring to a boil. Cook for 1 hour. Add salt and soy sauce.

27. Daikon Oroshi (grated radish)

1 Tbsp grated daikon	1 tsp sesame oil (boil
3 tsp soy sauce	and let cool)

Mix well. Serve individually at table.

28. Sautéed Onion

1 onion, cut mawashigiri	Pinch of salt
A little oil	

Sauté onion well. Cover and cook over low flame, waterless. Add salt. When ready to serve, sprinkle with green Nori.

29. Wild Vegetables

Sauté or cook in salt water and season vegetables with miso, salt, or soy sauce.

30. Vegetable Tempura

3" burdock root	1¼ cups water
½ carrot	½ tsp salt
1" lotus root	Oil
½" grated daikon	Soy sauce
1 cup whole wheat pastry flour	

Cut all vegetables sengiri. Mix flour and water and salt. Oil should be 3 inches deep in pan and heated to 350 degrees. When the batter-dipped vegetables are added to the oil, they should fall to the bottom of the pan and almost immediately float to the surface. Don't fry too many at a time as you won't get a nice crispy tempura. When a bit crisp on one side, turn over and crisp-up other side. Remove and drain well on a strainer pan and place on a paper towel to remove excess oil. Serve hot with grated daikon and soy sauce dip. Daikon is good for the digestion of fried food.

31. Koi-Koku (Carp soup)

1 lb carp	¾ cup miso
½ lb burdock, cut sasagaki	Used bancha tea leaves
(3 times as much burdock as	1 Tbsp sesame oil
carp when placed in pot)	1 piece ginger minced

Place 1 handful of used bancha tea leaves in a cotton bag and tie closed. Set aside. Remove bitter gall bladder (green or yellow colored) and cut whole carp into 1-inch slices (head, tail, scales, and bones). Sauté burdock until strong smell is gone. Add carp. Put tea bag on top of carp and cover with water 2 inches above carp. Simmer 4-5 hours, or until the bones become soft. Take out tea bag and add miso. Cook another 20 minutes. Add ginger. (If you use a pressure cooker, cook for 2 hours. Let pressure go down. Test to see if bones are soft. If not, continue cooking with pressure another hour. When tender, add miso and ginger.) Add more water as needed to cover carp 2 inches. Eat everything in the dish. Should you cut the gall bladder with your knife, immediately wash carp with hot bancha tea to remove the bitter taste; otherwise, you won't be able to eat the carp because the taste will be so bitter.

32. Aburage (Agé)

Put a dry kitchen towel on a cutting board. Cut tofu in half ⅓-inch thick. Cut each half into 4-5 pieces. Set tofu on the towel and cover with another cotton kitchen towel and another cutting board. Put a heavy book on top for pressure. Let set about 1 hour. Place 3 inches of oil in tempura pot. Heat oil until 350 degrees, add tofu and cook until golden color on one side, then turn over and brown on other side. Drain well in a strainer pan and place on a paper towel to remove any excess oil that may remain.

Use tofu that has been made with nigari. Nigari is a magnesium chloride that is left over by precipitation of NaCl. (See *Do of Cooking Vol. 1*, recipe 28.)

33. Deep-fried Vegetable Tofu (Ganmo)

1 lb tofu	2-3" jinenjo (nagaimo)
½" lotus root cut small	1-2" carrot cut small
2" burdock cut small	1 qt oil
1 cup whole wheat flour	

Remove tofu from soaking water. Grind well in a suribachi, adding a pinch of salt. Sauté vegetables in a skillet and add ground tofu. Grate jinenjo (nagaimo) and mix. Add a small amount of whole wheat flour to hold mixture together. Roll into small balls (like croquettes) and deep-fry until light brown on both sides.

34. Vegetable with Ganmo

5" daikon, cut ichogiri	1 med onion, cut mawashigiri
3" carrot, cut ¼" koguchi	Oil
3" burdock, cut ¼" koguchi	Water

Sauté burdock, onion, daikon, and carrot in that order. Sauté is in order from yin to yang, except for the burdock which is yang. (The reason that the burdock is sautéed first is that it contains a strong yin, potassium, in a high amount.) Add water to cover. Bring to a boil and add ganmo. Cook until tender. Add salt and soy sauce.

35. Dried Radish with Agé

½ cup dried (daikon) radish	Pinch of salt
2 onions, ½" mawashigiri cut	Water
5 agé (see recipe 32)	Soy sauce

Sauté onions. Wash and soak dried radish in water to cover for 20-30 minutes. Remove from soaking water. Reserve soaking water to use later. Sauté dried radish well. Add soaking water and cook. Add Agé and cook until tender. Add salt and soy sauce. Cook 30 minutes more.

36. Kenchin Soup

½ carrot, cut ⅛" koguchi	5 niboshi (dried fish)
3" daikon, cut ¼" ichogiri	minced (optional)
1 burdock root, cut ⅛" koguchi	1 Tbsp oil
½ bunch scallions, cut ¾"	3½ cups water
koguchi	5 taro, cut ⅛" koguchi

Sauté scallions and add Niboshi. Sauté until fish smell is gone. Add burdock, daikon, taro, and carrot. Sauté well. Add water to cover vegetables and a pinch of salt. Cook over medium heat about 1 hour. Season with salt and soy sauce or miso.

37. Deep-fried Wakame

Choose wakame that has no sand. Cut 2" x 3". Deep-fry in 2 inches of oil. Serve two or three pieces per person, with grated daikon and soy sauce. Variation: toast wakame over a flame, then crumble with fingers and sprinkle on rice.

38. Small Fish Nitsuke

25 pieces niboshi (iriko)	1-2 Tbsp soy sauce
Oil	

Deep-fry iriko until light yellow color. Boil soy sauce, add fried fish, and bring to a boil again. Shake pan up and down until all the juice is well-mixed. These can be kept for 1-2 years.

39. Omedeto (Congratulations! Cheers!)

⅔ cup rice   3⅔ cups water
⅓ cup aduki beans   Pinch of salt

Roast rice until golden brown. Cook with five times as much water until soft and creamy. Boil the beans in 1½ cups of water until tender, adding more water if necessary. Mix with rice and simmer 2-3 hours. Add salt.

If roasting rice for sick persons, use sesame oil in the pan. It gives a better taste. Add ⅓ cup roasted and ground sesame seeds and remove from flame.

If you use a pressure cooker, soak aduki beans overnight in four times as much water as beans. Add roasted rice and cook 40 minutes to 1 hour. Add salt and serve.

40. Yin/Yang Soboro

4" jinenjo grated   ½ cup miso
½ carrot minced   3 Tbsp oil
1" lotus root minced   1 tsp ginger minced
3 Tbsp goma (sesame seeds)

Sauté jinenjo and sesame seeds in oil. Add lotus root, carrot, and sauté well. Add miso. Cook over low flame like a tekka miso. Add ginger and cook as Tekka No. 1 (recipe 14).

41. Brown Rice Tea

⅓ cup rice   5 cups water
Pinch of salt

Roast rice to a light brown color. Add water and cook for 30 minutes. Add salt. Squeeze juice from rice using a cotton cloth bag. Residue left in cotton bag can be used in baking bread.

Replaces black or green tea.

42. Corn Meal

⅓ cup corn meal   Salt
1 tsp oil   1½ cups water

Sauté corn meal in oil about 5-10 minutes. Add water and cook for

30 minutes. Add salt. Should be like a thick porridge.

43. Tamari Bancha (syoban)

½ tsp soy sauce
⅓ cup bancha tea

Roast 3-year-old bancha leaves until a brown color. Combine 1 part tea to 10 parts water and bring to a boil. Let boil 10 to 15 minutes. Put soy sauce in a cup and add boiling bancha tea. Serve hot!

44. Umesho Bancha (salt plum tea)

½ cup bancha tea	1 small umeboshi plum
½ tsp soy sauce	2-3 drops ginger juice

Put mashed umeboshi plum, soy sauce, and ginger in a cup. Add boiling bancha tea and mix. Drink and eat all except the seed of the plum. For children, don't use ginger. Add 1 teaspoon of kuzu instead. It is easier for them to drink. Dissolve kuzu in cold water before adding it to the tea. Cook a few minutes until kuzu cooks clear in the tea.

45. Daikon Tea No. 1

3 Tbsp daikon grated	1 tsp ginger grated and squeezed for juice
1 Tbsp soy sauce	2-3 cups bancha tea

Mix daikon, ginger juice, and soy sauce in a bowl. Add boiling bancha tea. Serve hot. Use once only. Drink hot when in bed to keep your body warm.

46. Daikon Tea No. 2

1½" daikon, grate and	3 Tbsp warm water
squeeze out juice = 1 Tbsp	Pinch of salt

Mix daikon juice and water. Bring to a boil, add salt, and serve. Never use raw daikon juice as it is very yin. Drink only once a day.

47. Mugwort Tea (yomogi or armoise)

Add ⅔ cup water to 1-2 tiny pieces of mugwort. Cook 10 minutes and add salt and serve.

48. Scallion Miso

2 bunches scallion, cut ⅓" koguchi	2 heaping Tbsp mugi miso 1-2 Tbsp sesame oil

Mince scallion roots. Heat oil and sauté roots for a few minutes. Add green parts until color changes. Add white part. Sauté a few minutes more, add miso, and cook covered for 5 minutes. Mix well and serve.

49. Onion Miso

1 cup onions, cut ¼" mawashigiri	1 Tbsp oil 1-2 heaping Tbsp mugi miso

Heat pan and sauté onions in oil until transparent. Add miso and cook with cover on until miso has a fragrant smell. Use once or twice a day.

50. Shigure Miso

¾ cup lotus root, minced	4 Tbsp sesame oil
¾ cup onions, minced	1½ cups mugi miso
¼ cup burdock root, minced	1 cup water
¼ cup carrots, minced	1 Tbsp tahini
1 tsp ginger, minced	

Mince all the vegetables separately in very fine pieces. Heat oil in thick iron pan. Sauté the burdock about 5 minutes until strong smell is gone. Then add onions and sauté 5 minutes, add lotus root and stir two or three times, add carrots and sauté a few minutes, and add ⅓ cup water and bring to a boil. Cover and cook on medium flame for 5 minutes. Mix miso with ½ cup water, add to vegetables, bring to boil, and then cook 40 minutes covered on low flame. Stir gently, add ginger, and cook 30 minutes; add tahini and cook 5 more minutes, then take off cover for 10 minutes and cook until excess liquid is evaporated.

Shigure Miso is more yin than Tekka Miso because water is used in its preparation. It doesn't keep as long as Tekka. Reheat between uses to keep from spoiling. Good with rice cream, oatmeal, toasted bread, and as a side dish with rice balls.

51. Pheasant Nitsuke No. 1

Whole pheasant   ⅔-1 cup mugi miso
3 Tbsp sesame oil   5 Tbsp ginger minced

Twist newspaper like a ball. Fire this paper and burn the pheasant's hair with this fire. Wash thoroughly and towel dry. Place breast down, uncovered, on a rack in a shallow roasting pan. Preheat oven to 300 degrees and bake for 40 minutes to 1 hour. Use sliced meat only. Chop it into small pieces. Heat oil and sauté ginger 5 minutes, add meat and sauté well, add miso and stir gently, and cook until miso has a fragrant smell.

52. Pheasant Nitsuke No. 2

Whole pheasant, roasted   3 Tbsp sesame oil
  as in recipe 51   1–1½ cups soy sauce
¼ cup ginger sliced thin

Take off skin, use meat only, and slice very thin. Heat oil and sauté ginger a few minutes. Add meat and sauté on a high flame until all juice is gone. Add soy sauce. Cook on medium flame with cover for 20 minutes, then turn over and cook 10 more minutes. Take off cover and turn to a high flame, shaking pan until excess liquid is evaporated.

This dish (like preserves) keeps for a long time. Use in noodle soup, fried rice, noodle sauce, etc. George Ohsawa gave me this recipe when I cooked pheasant for the first time in Chico.

Bouillon

Bones from whole pheasant   ⅓ cup parsley chopped
1 small onion   10 cups water
1 small carrot

Break or chop pheasant bones into 2- to 3-inch pieces. Add water and bring to a boil without cover. Lower flame, continue to boil, and skim off scum. When stock is clear, add carrot, onion, and parsley. Continue cooking about 3 hours until about 6 cups of stock remain. Strain and use stock for cooking.

53. Chrysanthemum Tea

Place 3 medium-sized fresh green leaves in 1 cup of water. Let boil 15 minutes or until the volume is reduced to ⅔ cup.

54. Brown Rice Soup

1 cup brown rice	10 cups water
Pinch of salt	

Roast rice until well-browned. Heat rice and water until it reaches a rapid boil. Then add salt and reduce volume to one-half.

55. Rice Coffee

¼ cup brown rice   3½ cups water

Roast the rice till golden. Add the water and boil for 20 minutes. Strain and serve.

In winter, add a drop of soy sauce to make a good pick-up drink.

56. Kokkoh

4 cups brown rice	1½ cups oat groats
2 cups sweet brown rice	¾ cup brown sesame seeds

Wash and drain ingredients. Lightly roast each separately. Grind to flour consistency. Best when freshly roasted and ground. Refrigerate in closed container if storing long. (See *Chico-San Cookbook*, 7-J for uses.)

57. Kuzu

Cook kuzu with enough water to make a thin soup consistency. Season with salt or soy sauce and serve hot.

58. Umesho Kuzu

1 umeboshi plum separated into pieces	2 cups water
1 heaping tsp kuzu mixed with 2 Tbsp water	5-6 drops ginger juice, grate ginger and squeeze out juice
	2 tsp soy sauce

Bring umeboshi plum and water to a boil without cover. Add dissolved kuzu, cook 15 minutes without cover until slightly thick. Add soy sauce and bring to a boil; add ginger juice and bring to a boil. Serve immediately.

59. Bajra (a variety of millet)

⅓ cup bajra   Salt
1 tsp oil   1½ cups water

Sauté bajra in oil about 5-10 minutes. Add water and cook for 30 minutes. Add salt. Should be like a thick porridge.

60. Shio Kombu

8 oz kombu   1 qt soy sauce

Clean kombu, by wiping it with a damp cloth, and cut into ½-inch squares. Allow to dry on absorbent paper. Soak overnight in soy sauce to cover.

Put kombu and soy sauce into a pot, cover, and bring to a boil. Lower flame and simmer about 3 hours, stirring occasionally. Remove cover and mix thoroughly. Continue cooking and stirring until soy sauce liquid cooks away. These are extremely salty and only 2 or 3 should be eaten at any one meal. They can be stored in a covered container for many months. This kombu is good inside rice balls instead of umeboshi.

61. Mochi

Mochi is made from sweet brown rice that is cooked, steamed, and pounded. It has been favored by Japanese and other Asian people for a long time as a treat, snack, party food, or confection.

The steaming and pounding make mochi easy to digest. So it is a good food for someone with a weak stomach or intestines. It is very tasty, which makes it an ideal snack for growing children who often ask for a treat between meals. Mochi tastes good in the summertime when one loses appetite due to the heat.

Mochi holds yang energy from the pounding so it is considered to be a food that increases stamina. Japanese laborers and farmers often eat mochi. In the winter, the farmers make it from freshly milled sweet rice and rice flour.

Pregnant women eat mochi often so that their baby will show durability after birth. The mochi helps build elasticity in muscles. Nursing mothers eat mochi to ensure a plentiful milk supply.

If mochi is adopted in this country in the same way French pastry and Chinese food have been, it will bring delight to American meals while building healthier and happier families.

    5 cups sweet brown rice   7 cups sweet brown rice flour
    5 cups water

Rinse rice and soak for 24 hours. Put in pressure cooker and let pressure come up to full, then cook at low heat 20 minutes. Turn off and let stand on stove 40-50 minutes. Mix flour with hot rice and pound with a wooden hammer. Wet both hands in cold water, and mash rice by pressing firmly in a flat pan until all rice grains are thoroughly mashed. Bring water to boil in a steamer pan. Put a wet cloth into the pan and place raw mochi on top. Cover with the same cloth. Cook at a high heat for 20 minutes. Pierce mochi with a dry chopstick. If nothing sticks to it when it is withdrawn, mochi is done. Mochi is usually shaped into 3-inch flat rounds.

62. Special Rice Soup

    1 cup brown rice   Pinch of salt
    7 cups water   1 tsp sesame oil

Fry rice in sesame oil until browned. Add water and salt and bring to a boil. Cook with cover until rice is soft. Do not stir. Eat as thick soup.

63. Aduki Bean Soup

    1 handful aduki beans   1½ qts water
    Pinch of salt

Boil aduki beans in water, adding more water as needed, and salt only when the beans are completely soft and foamy. Ordinarily, cooking takes 4 hours but adding a couple of square inches of kombu reduces cooking time to ½ hour.

64. Lotus Root Tea (dried or fresh)

1½" lotus root grated = 1 Tbsp   2-3 drops ginger juice
½ cup boiling water   Pinch of salt

Grate the raw lotus root and squeeze juice through a cheesecloth. Add water and ginger juice to lotus root juice. Simmer gently. Add salt and serve.

65. Bancha Tea (3-year-old tea)

Roast the leaves until they turn brown in color. If used for medication, boil leaves 15 minutes. If for daily use with meals, add 1-2 tablespoons of tea leaves to 4 cups of boiling water. Steep a few minutes and serve. Keep leftover tea in a porcelain, earthenware, or glass jar. Add water to leaves and cook 15 minutes for second use. Just before serving, add a pinch of fresh leaves for a fresher flavor. Continue making tea in this way until the leaves stack up about 1 inch in the bottom of the tea kettle. Then start with new leaves again.

This tea grows on the coast of Japan, getting fresh sea air.

66. Ranshyo

1 egg   Soy sauce (½ of half an eggshell full)

Beat egg until frothy peaks form. Add soy sauce and mix well. Drink before bedtime. Take once a day only! Do not drink this more than 3 days in a row.

67. Gomashio (sesame salt)

Adult (strong):   Child or Senior:
8-12 Tbsp sesame seeds   12-16 Tbsp sesame seeds
   (unhulled black)   (unhulled black)
1 Tbsp salt   1 Tbsp salt

Roast the salt in a dry pan, stirring constantly until the acid smell is gone, and grind in a suribachi. Wash sesame seeds well. Drain. Roast seeds at medium heat. Stir constantly with one hand while shaking the pan frequently with the other, until they are slightly roasted and begin to jump about in pan. Test by trying to mash a seed between fourth finger and thumb. If it mashes easily, they are done. Put seeds inside suribachi with the ground salt, grind together until seeds are half-crushed.

Don't grind too much. Grind lightly and take your time.

It may be necessary to vary the adult proportions as well as child's, as the amount of salt required varies with each individual. Best not to use with a large amount of salt. Never make more than 1 week's supply, and always store in tightly-closed container. (Also see *Do of Cooking Vol. 2*, recipe 100.)

68. Yannoh

3 cups brown rice	2 cups chick peas
2½ cups wheat berries	1 cup chicory root
1½ cups aduki beans	

Wash all the ingredients and allow to drain. Roast them separately until dark brown. Be careful with the chick peas as they burn easily. Combine, and grind very finely. (See *Chico-San Cookbook,* 7-J for uses.)

Procedures for External Treatment

69. Ginger Compress

⅓ cup grated ginger   10 cups boiled water

Put grated ginger in a cotton cloth bag and tie. Place in hot water until water turns yellow, then squeeze ginger juice into water. Keep the water hot, but don't boil as boiling kills the effectiveness of the ginger. Dip a towel or cotton cloth in this water and squeeze out excess water. Put this hot cloth over painful area. Cover with two dry flannel cloths and top with a sheet of plastic to keep towel warm as long as possible. When it cools, repeat. Use three or four times a day, 20 minutes each time. Change to fresh ginger water each day of use. (See illustrations that follow.)

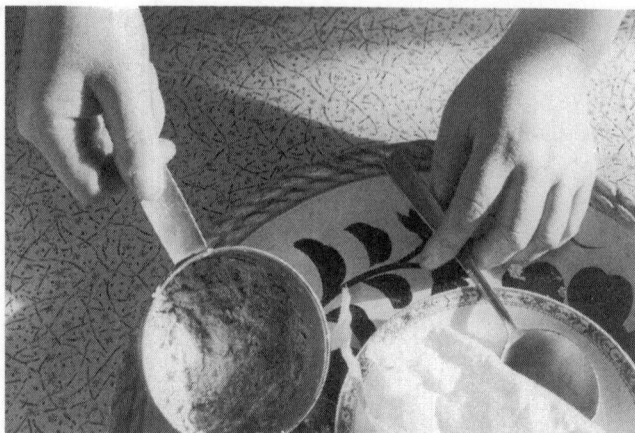

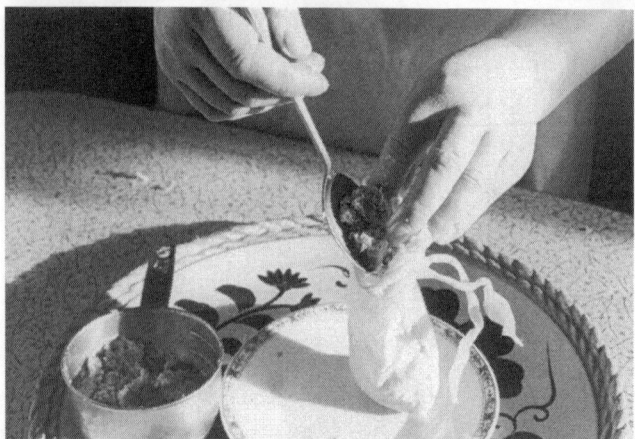

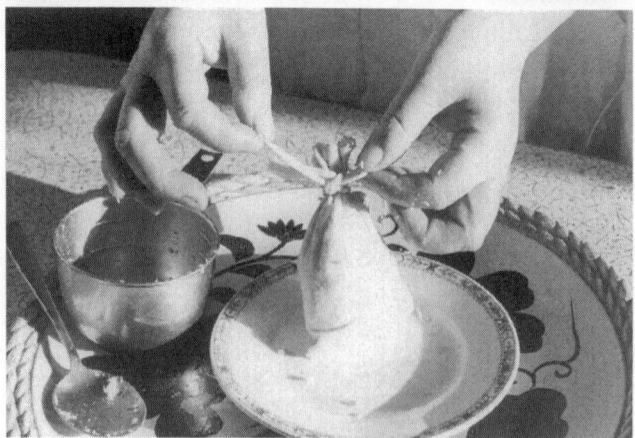

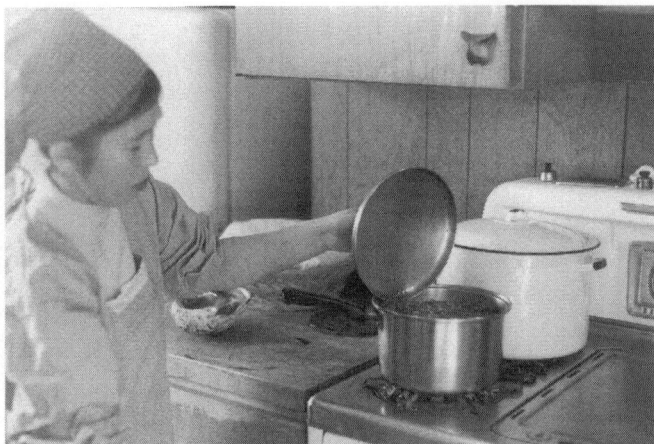

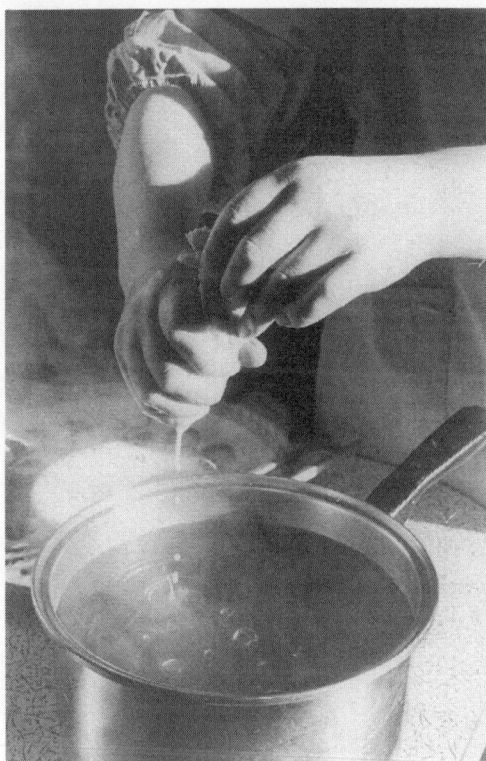

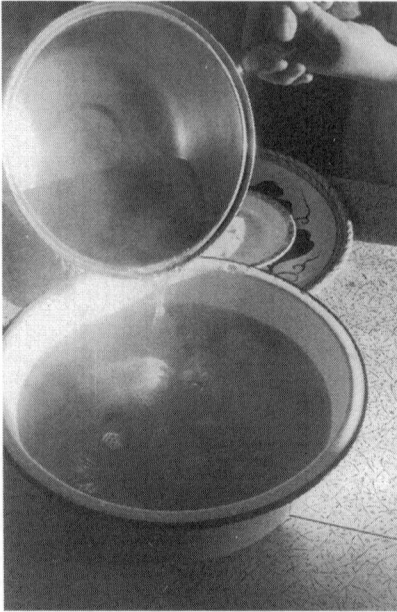
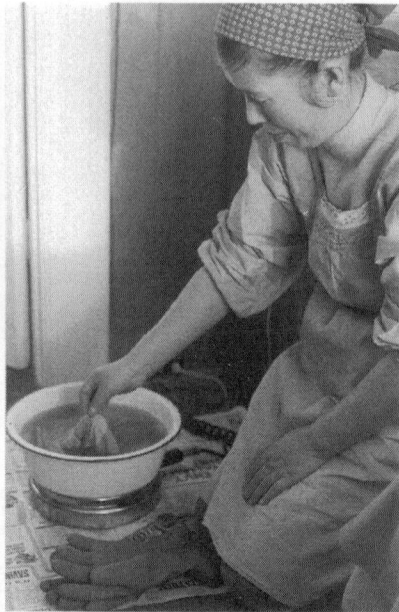
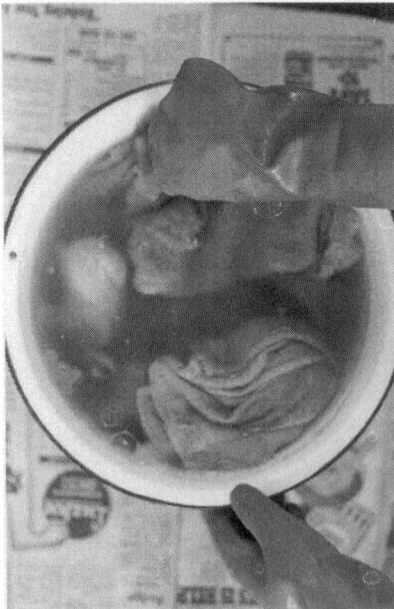
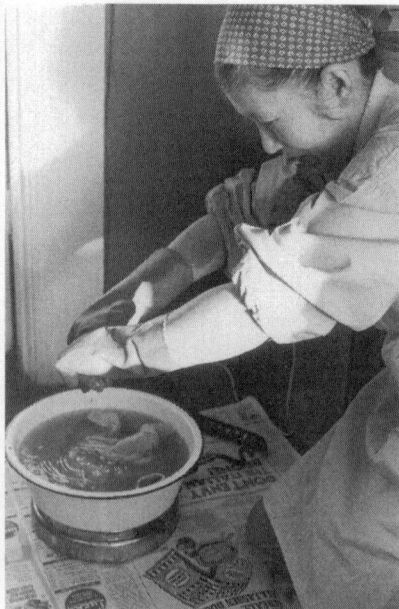

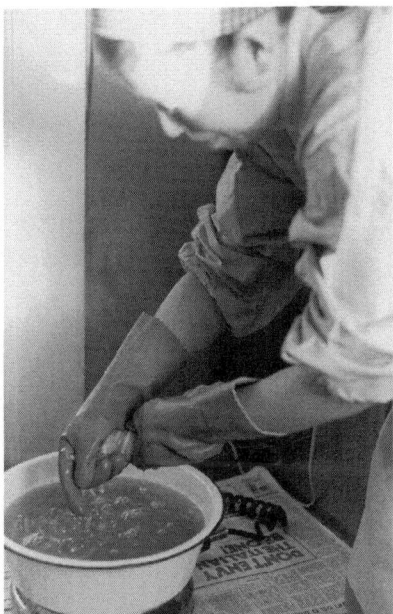
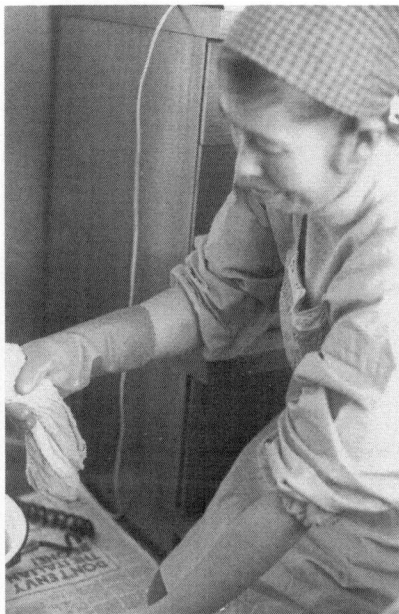
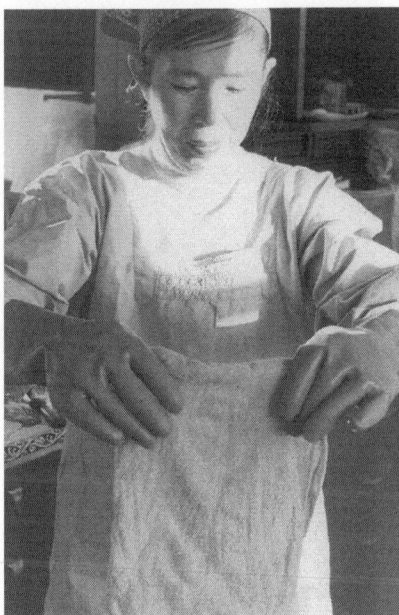
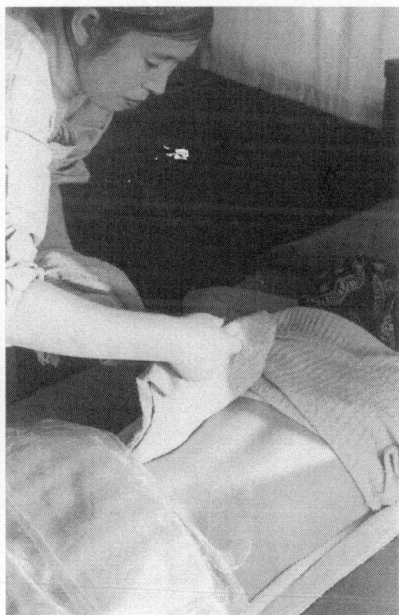

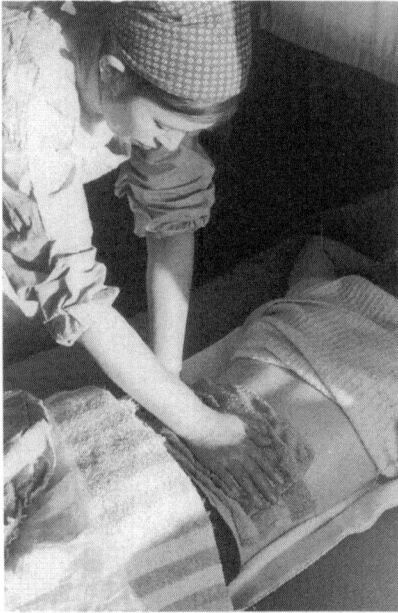
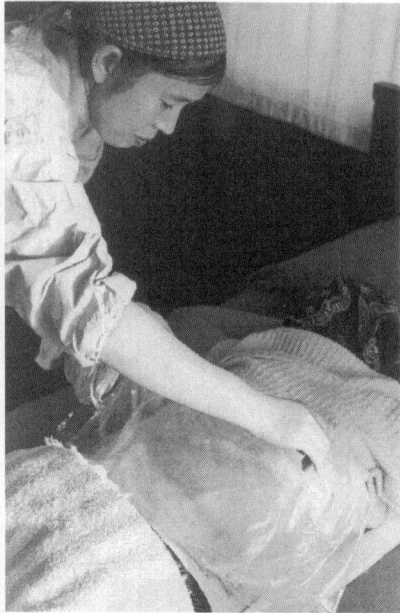
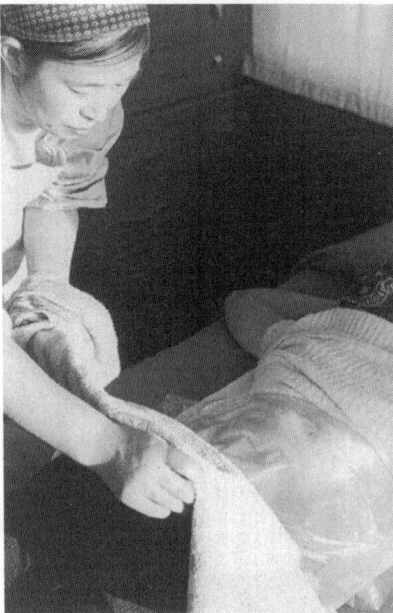
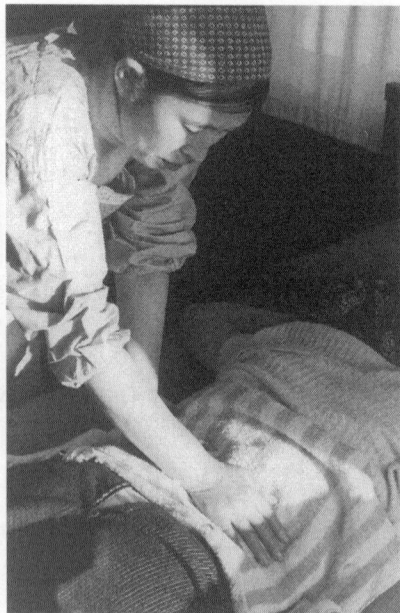

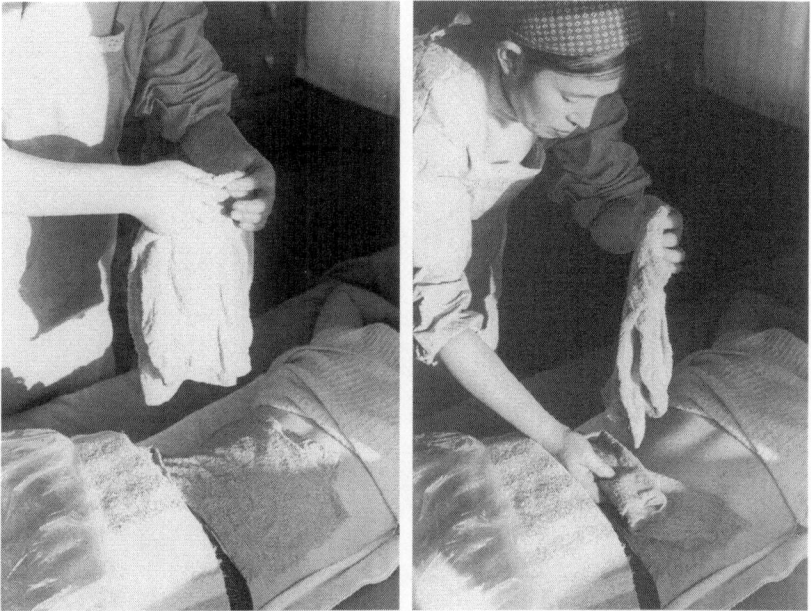

70. Albi Plaster

 Albi (taro)
 Ginger
 White or whole wheat flour

Wash a small taro and take off skin and grate. Grate ginger, using
1/10th the amount of taro. Mix taro and ginger and add flour to equal
the amount of taro used. Mix. Spread on a flannel cloth ½ inch thick
and place on the injured part. Keep on 4 or 5 hours. Then change to a
new taro plaster. Before and after the taro plaster is applied, a ginger
compress can be used. Cover the taro plaster with gauze for protec-
tion, wrap the gauze around the part of the body to which the plaster
is applied so that it does not slip away. (See illustrations that follow.)

Albi Powder: Dry albi and ginger and grind to a fine powder. Mix in
proportions of 1 to 10 (ginger to albi). Keep this ready to make albi
plasters.

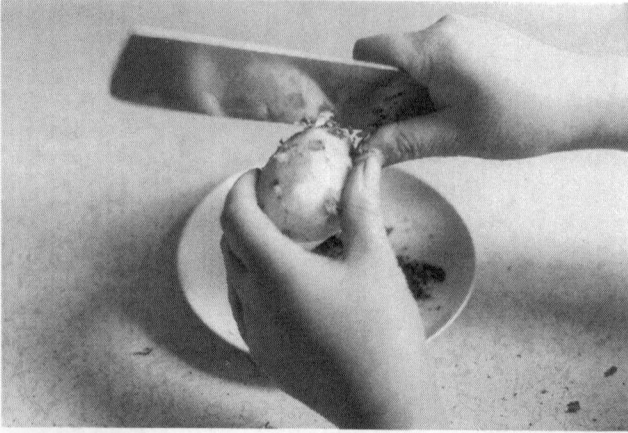

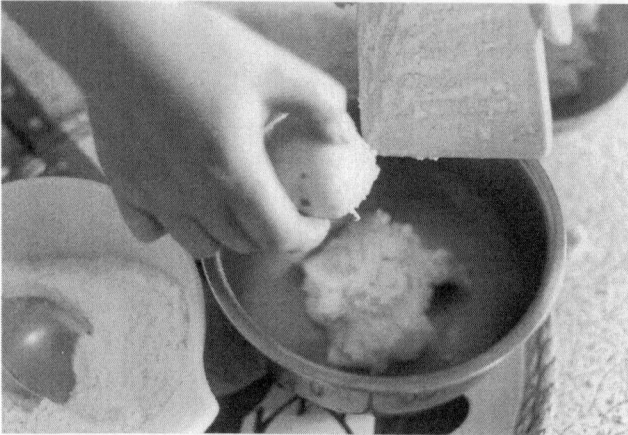

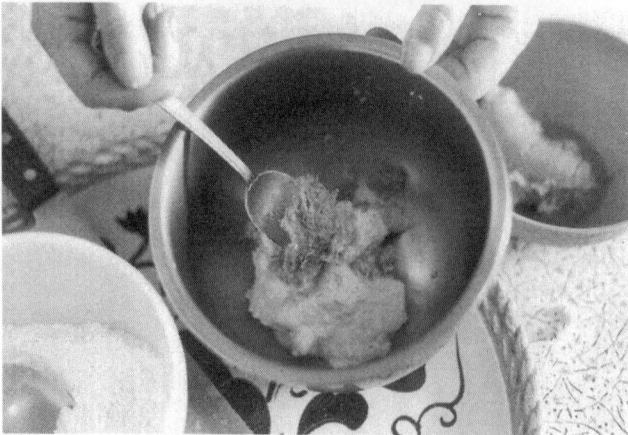

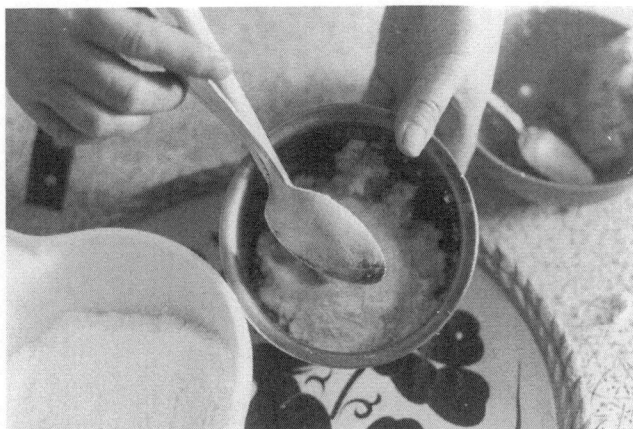

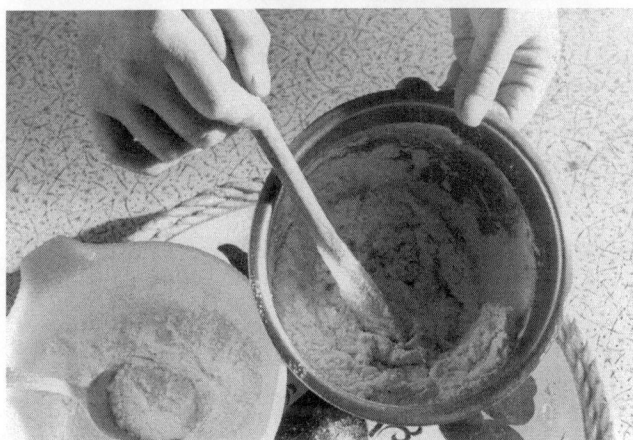

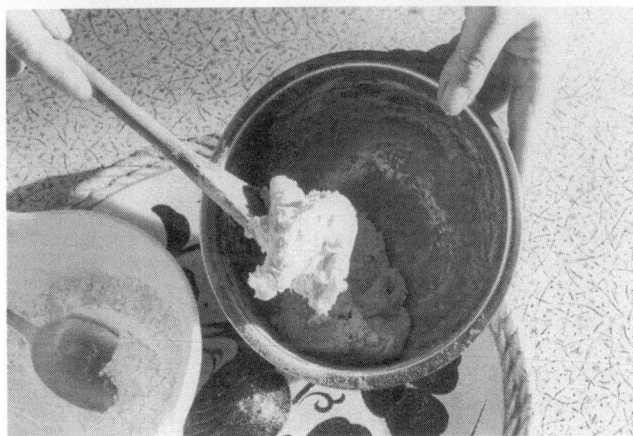

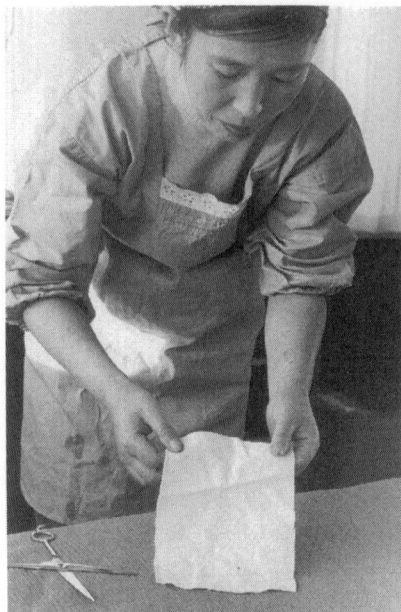
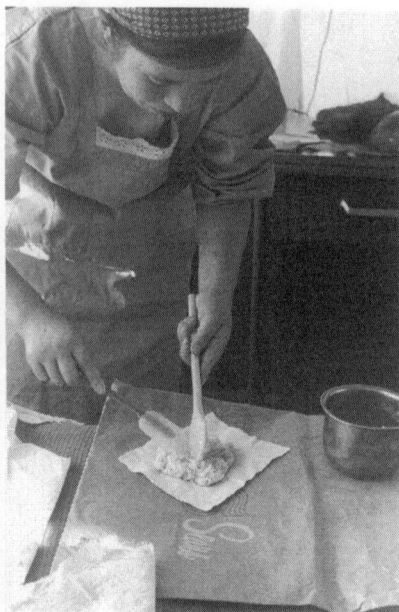
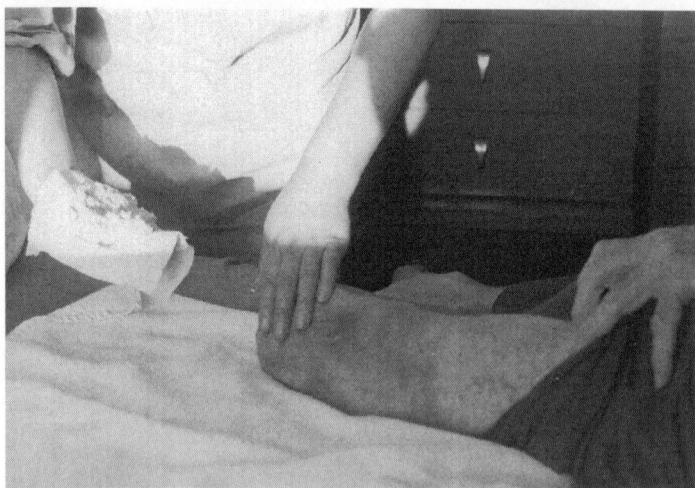

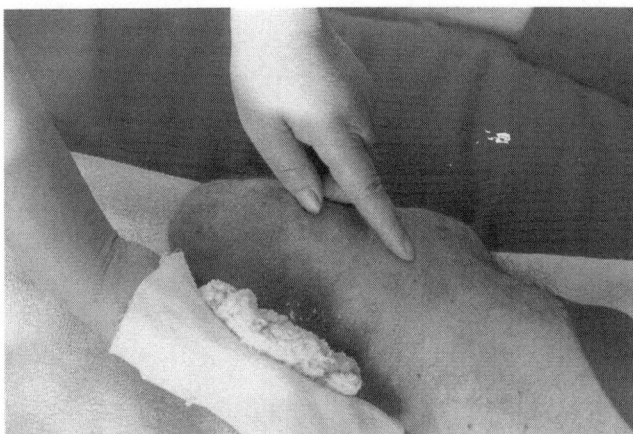

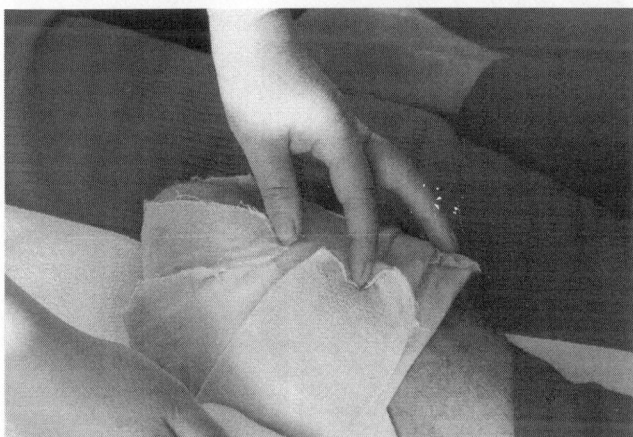

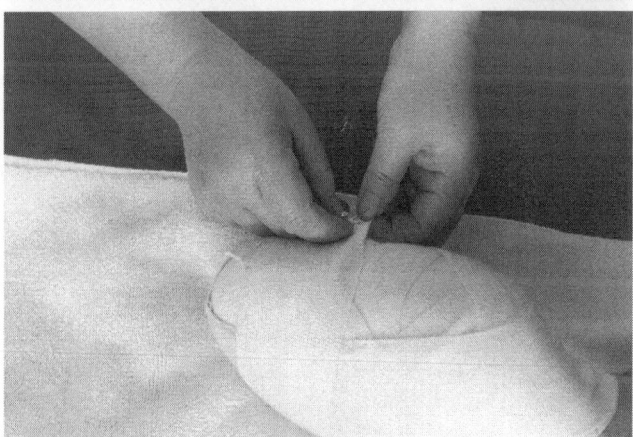

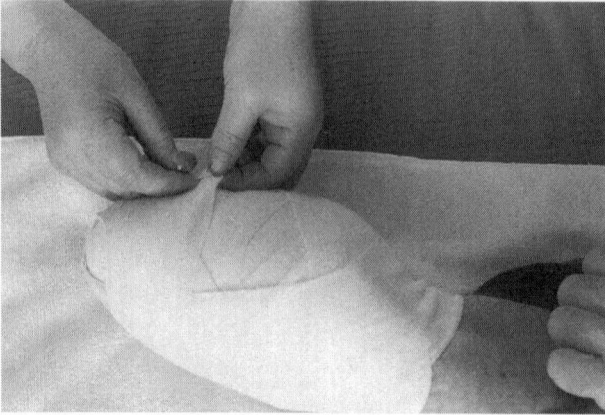

71. Tofu Plaster

Tofu or soybeans   White or whole wheat flour
Ginger

Soak raw soybeans till soft and mash; or squeeze water from tofu and mash. Add 10-20 percent flour. Grate a small ginger and add. Place the plaster on the injured or affected part, cover with a cotton cloth (NEVER cover with synthetic material) and use a gauze wrapper as above (albi plaster). Apply to head or neck only. Never below the neck. Check body temperature frequently so that it doesn't drop too low.

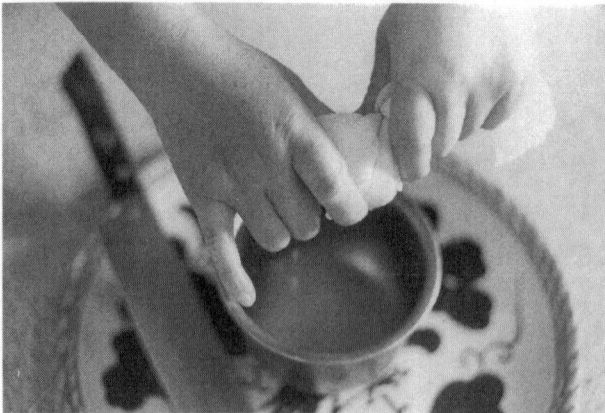

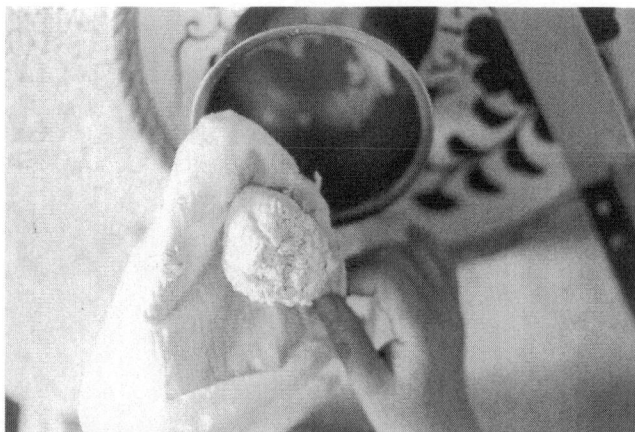

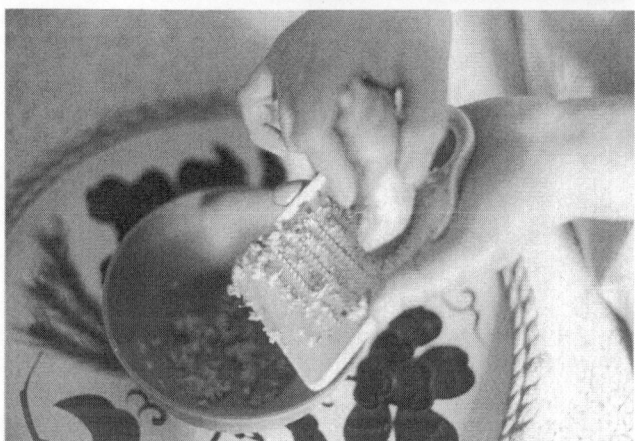

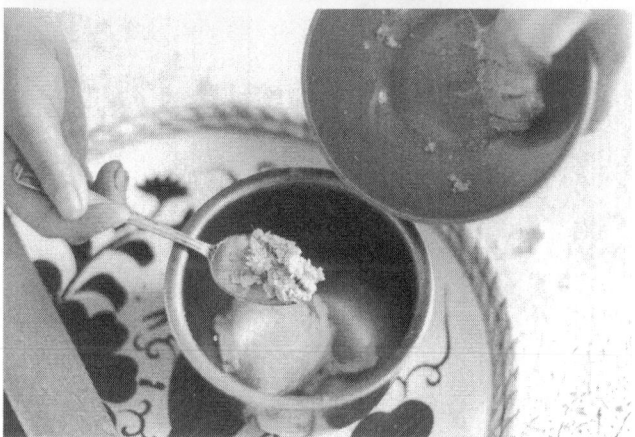

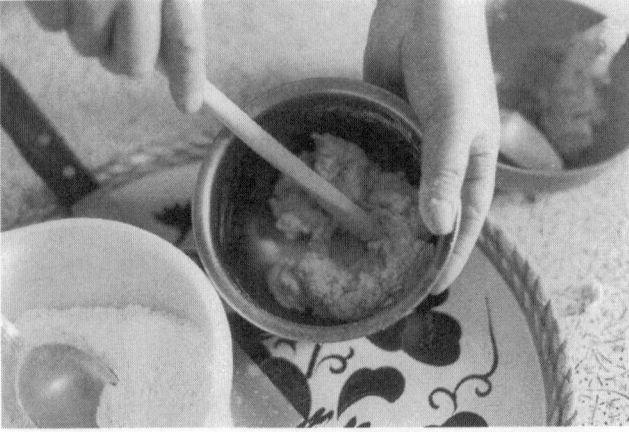

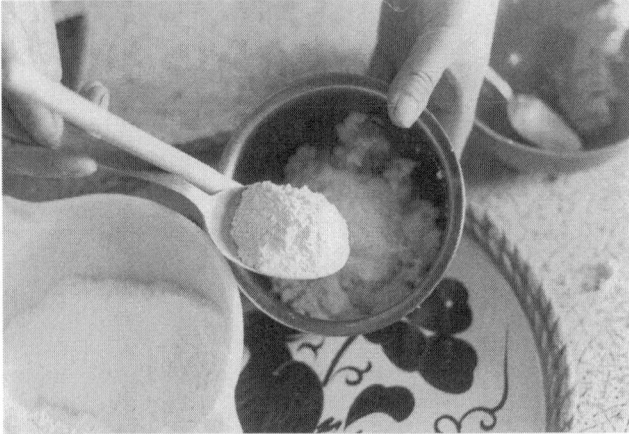

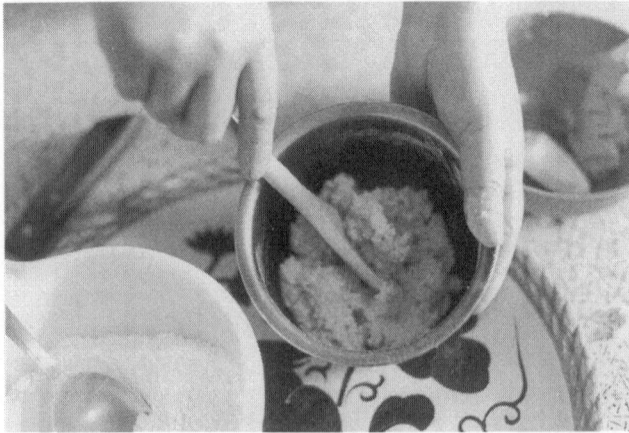

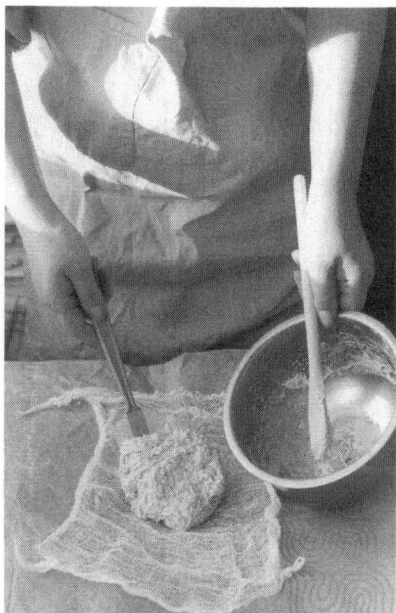
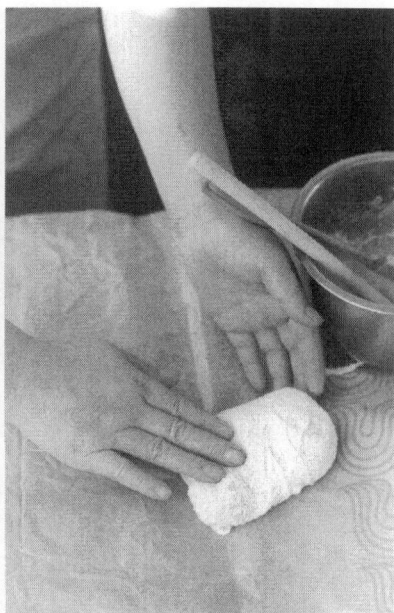
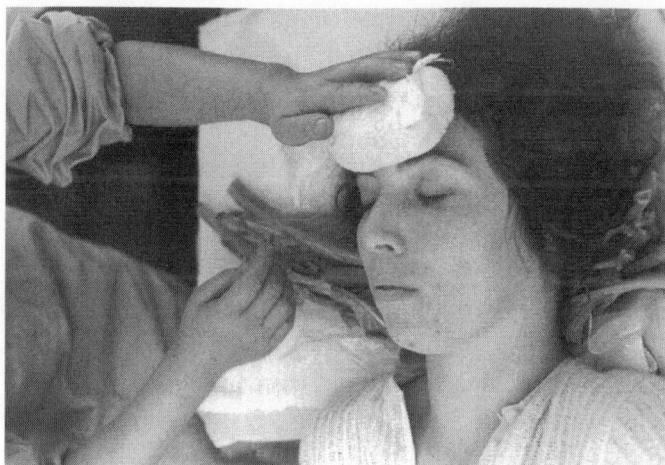

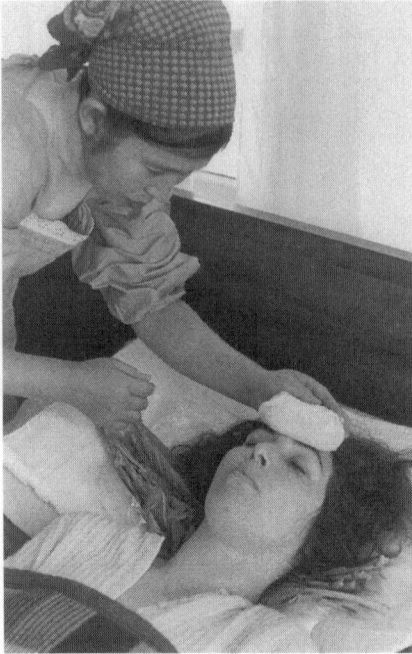

72. Carp Plaster

Carp   Flour

Use live carp. Hit the living carp's head two or three times. Chop the head off with a knife and grind well. Add a bit of flour and spread on oiled paper, or on waxed paper. Apply to the injured part. In cases of acute pneumonia, give 1 tablespoon of carp's blood, which is taken from the freshly-killed carp. Open the chest and reserve the blood in a small dish. At the same time, apply the carp plaster over the back as well as chest areas. Take sick person's temperature every 30 minutes. As soon as the temperature reaches normal, remove the plaster.

Blood should be taken only from freshly-killed carp, although meat from other fresh carp may be used in the plaster. If carp is unavailable, use hamburger or other fatty meat in the plaster.

73. Soba Plaster

Buckwheat flour
Warm water

Mix flour with enough water tomake a paste and spread on a flannel cloth. Apply to injured part.

74. Sesame Oil

Bring sesame oil to a boil. Filter through a Red Cross cotton bandage. Using eye-dropper, apply only one drop.

75. Hibayu

4-5 bunches hiba
20 cups water
1 handful salt

Hiba is made of daikon leaves dried in the shade.

Bring hiba to boil in water and cook 30-60 minutes: Add salt. This is good for a hip bath before bedtime, immersing hip bone 8-10 inches above the knee. The hotter the better but do not burn yourself. Sit in this for 15-20 minutes. When you start to sweat, dry off and keep warm. Go to bed immediately. Do this each night.

76. Sesame Oil and Ginger

Mix thoroughly equal parts ginger juice and sesame oil. Shake to make an emulsion. Rub directly on the head for all headaches, dandruff, and loss of hair. A drop of this emulsion in the ear helps middle ear inflammation.

77. Apple Juice

Grate apple and squeeze through cheesecloth.

78. Radish Juice

Grate daikon radish and squeeze through cheesecloth. Use juice only.

79. Salt Compress

Heat salt and place in a pillowcase.

80. Dentie

Eggplant   Salt

Preserve calyx (head) of eggplant with 20 percent salt in a closed crock (jar) under pressure for several years. Then dry and char. Massage gums 5 minutes with this ash to cure any child's toothache. For pyorrhea, brush teeth and rinse your mouth; then rub a pinch of dentie on the outer gums; close your mouth until gums absorb the black powder.

81. Nukayu

Rice bran   Water

Put 4 handfuls of rice bran in a cotton bag and boil in 3 quarts of water.

82. Chlorophyll Plaster

Any leafy greens   Dry peppermint

Pound greens to a paste, adding 10 percent peppermint. Place directly on forehead or on any inflamed part of the body. Use in place of albi plaster when albi is not available.

83. Hot Foot Bath

Put very hot water in a big pan and place feet in for 10 minutes.

84. Green Leaves Application

The leaves of any green leafy vegetable such as kale, collards, mustard greens, or any wild plant can be used directly on an affected area. For cooling relief from fever, the greens may be placed at the back of the neck while lying down (see illustrations that follow). Secure with a bandage if needed.

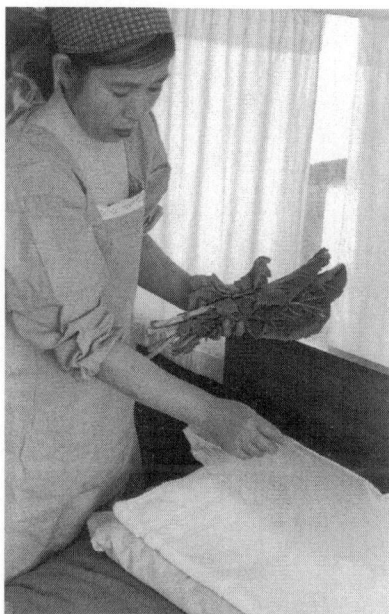
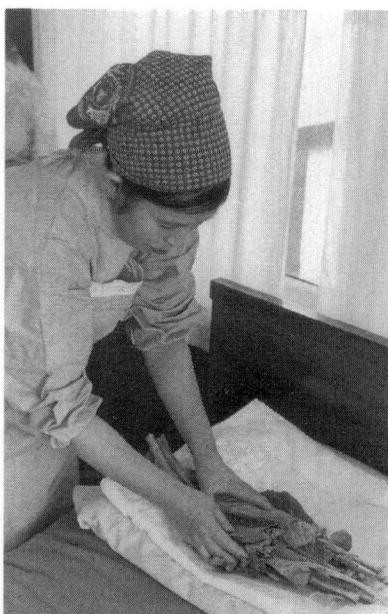

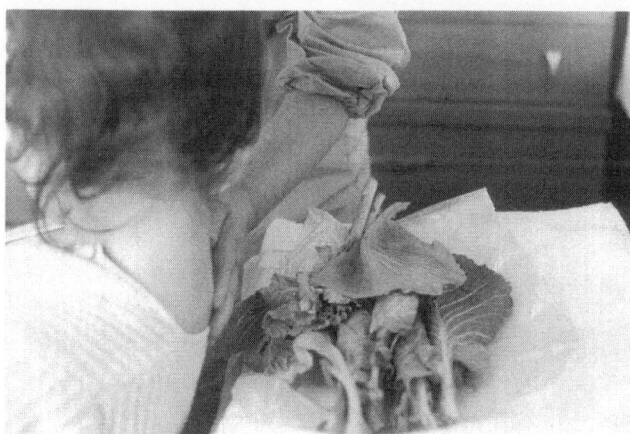

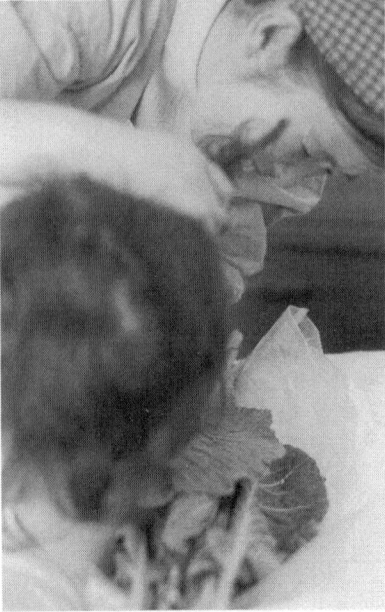
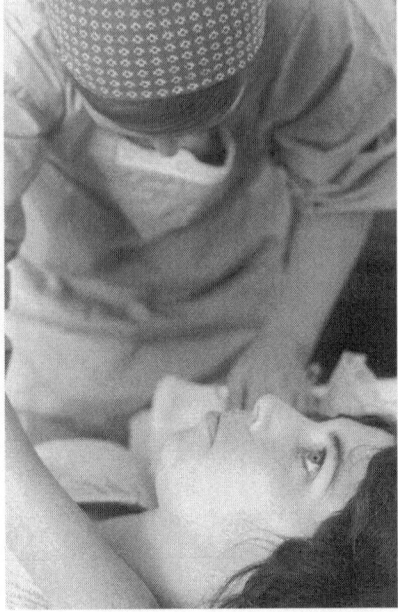

Macrobiotic Remedies

Sicknesses are discussed according to the area of the body affected:

A. Head and Brain

B. Eyes

C. Ears

D. Nose

E. Mouth

F. Face

G. Throat

H. Neck and Shoulders

I. Chest

J. Abdomen

K. Legs

L. Whole Body

M. Cravings, Habits and Addictions

N. Infections

Any sicknesses not discussed here may be treated by macrobiotic healers who have a deeper understanding of ayurvedic medicine.

In cooking for sick people especially, you must prepare food that is delicious and aesthetically appealing. Cooking is the art of life and of creation. The real artist knows how to create freedom and peace: biological, physiological and social freedom, and peace.

First, see that the food is appetizing. Do not use chemically treated ingredients or cooking utensils. Almost all commercially available oils contain preservatives. Avoid chemically fertilized or sprayed vegetables. Except for special medicines and foods, try to use vegetables grown within a 500-mile radius. Do not use imported products except for certain foods that are not available in this country. In this age of capitalism and mercantilist free-exchange, most farm businesses, plantations, and garden farms use chemical products the same as do factories.

Become a master in the art of cooking. Cook with love. To become a true artist, you can start with theory or practice—I suggest the latter. Theory will follow by itself. Work day-by-day. Your patient is your judge and jury. If he is satisfied and is getting healthier everyday by eating your cooking, then you too are getting healthier.

In Japan, there are schools of traditional cooking. Some teachers there can take a common food like soybeans or buckwheat flour and prepare hundreds of different dishes with them. They cook good food constantly, taking into consideration the situation at hand: the season, the age and original constitution of their patient, the physical surroundings, and his activities—so that their patients never get sick. The highest dream of a good cook is health, longevity, and Supreme Judgment (clear, just-thinking in harmony with the Order of the Universe)—which, after all, should be the highest goal of all science and philosophy.

The art of cooking in Buddhism reached its highest level hundreds of years ago in China and Japan, though today it is almost forgotten after 80 years of indoctrination in Western nutrition.

When cooking for yourself and others, you will undoubtedly wonder why I suggest vegetables like onions and lotus root cooked with salt and oil but little water, why other foods are totally forbidden (like sugar, tomatoes, potatoes, eggplant, animal products, and fruit) for most sick people beginning the diet. This is because most sicknesses today are caused by excess yin.

For our yang ancestors, leafy green vegetables and fruit may have been good medicine, but they are not suitable for people with yin constitutions. Root vegetables are best for restoring man's health today.

Tomatoes, potatoes, eggplant, relatively recently introduced from tropical climates to temperate ones, are as foreign to our constitutions as animal foods or chemical and industrial products. This will become clearer to you as you understand more deeply the biological and physiological basis of Far Eastern philosophy.

There's no danger in trying my suggestions for a week. You may then want to continue further.

[Editor's Note: You may panic at the seemingly indiscriminate recommendation of gomasio and narrow eating—don't! All the following treatments are short-term, to be discontinued when the reactions are reversed, and naturally subject to common-sense judgment and yin/yang diagnosis of the particular case at hand.]

A. Head and Brain

Baldness:

Follow the procedural instructions and your loss of hair will stop. On the average, you lose 10 hairs daily. The life of an eyebrow is several months, an eyelash several weeks. Everything is constantly changing—all you have to do is find the right leaven in your food and you can direct your own change: your lethargy, harsh voice, pouting expression, clumsiness, even your moodiness. If you are skeptical, eat some fruit, a tomato, an eggplant after eating well a couple of weeks: the following day you'll lose 10 times the amount of hair. Then use the specific external treatment (equal parts sesame oil and ginger juice). In six months your scalp will have put out a luxuriant new growth. If not, then your sickness is very deep-rooted, you have overeaten too long, or you haven't followed the preliminary suggestions carefully enough. Please don't give up though, becuase one of the most important organs—your heart—is at stake.

Encephalitic Meningitis:

One teaspoon gomasio at each meal. Shave the head. Apply ginger compresses five times a day, ½ hour each time. Then apply albi plaster every 4 hours.

Epilepsy:

There are yin and yang epilepsies. Yin is caused by excess yin food intake, and yang is caused by excess yang food intake.

Both cause constipation at the start of the disease. A yang seizure is tight and contracted (rigid and stiff) or violent. A yin seizure is a lapse of consciousness, a slump, or coma. At the beginning of a seizure, a patient may be lock-jawed or unconscious. At that time, you cannot give any medicines, so massage the stomach gently to help relax the intestines and calm the patient down.

Yang seizure is accompanied by eyes looking straight ahead. In a yin seizure, the eyes are up in the head (extremely sanpaku), and hands are open.

In a yang seizure, when the patient wakes up, give him fresh apple juice, made by grating an apple and squeezing 1 cup of the juice through a cotton cloth.

In a yin seizure, give umesho bancha (see recipe 44). To prevent yin seizures, serve 1 teaspoon of gomasio at each meal, sprinkled on the food. If you feel a seizure coming on, take 1 teaspoon of gomasio. If you crave more salt, take 1 teaspoon tekka (see recipes 14, 15, 16) or fried miso in addition to the gomasio.

Hair-Greying or Falling Out:

Greying is caused by excess yang, and falling hair is caused by excess yin. Follow preliminary diet and also refer to "Baldness.

Headaches:

Chronic headaches, whether recurrent or constant, are signals of very serious danger, especially in the case of migraines. Follow, very strictly, the preliminary suggestions. A common headache may be relieved by rubbing sesame oil and ginger on the forehead. (See recipe 76.)

Idiocy, Imbecility, Neurasthenia:

Very strict adherence to the preliminary suggestions cures these sicknesses. Three years ago, several well-known public and private institutions for mental diseases in Japan adopted the macrobiotic way of eating. If you are unable to cure these diseases, then you are handcuffed in any effort to eliminate crime, poverty, war. War is the most serious sin committed by well-masked "adult" idiots, imbeciles, weak-brained people. We eat; therefore, we think, see, move, walk, love, quarrel, kill, steal, cheat—in harmony or in discord with the Order of the Universe.

Insomnia:
Preliminary diet with a teaspoon of gomasio before going to bed. Also try hot foot bath (see recipe 83) 15 minutes before going to sleep.

Schizophrenia and Psychological Estrangement:
There are two different kinds of mental disease: excessive yang and excessive yin.

Symptoms of the first are loudness, violence, irritability, meanness (the radjasic characteristics). Signs of the second are withdrawal and lethargy (tamasic traits). A diet with more yin foods (rich in vitamin C and a high potassium/sodium ratio) will cure the first kind. Yang foods such as lotus root, lily tubers, pumpkin, or the preliminary diet with a little gomasio added are indicated for treating the second kind.

Proper yin/yang balance ranges from 5 parts potassium to 1 part sodium up to 7:1 or even 10:1, determined by dry weight. Consider the following: tomatoes 230:3, potatoes 410:6, eggplant 220:5, mushrooms 57.2:7.6, grapes 250:6, bamboo shoots 62.5:4.2, nuts 450:2, plums 600:5. These foods are obviously disastrous for a person with a basically yin constitution or somebody in a very yinnized condition.

Both excess yin and excess yang may be brought back into proportion by following the preliminary diet. Aggressiveness and sleepwalking can be eliminated by eating more yin foods or foods prepared in a more yin fashion. Weakness and hysteria by more yang or simply well-balanced cooking.

Sleeping Sickness:
The only cure is strict adherence to the preliminary diet. This disease is carried by a virus of unknown origin, perhaps strengthened by radioactivity. An already intoxicated state may further a person's

vulnerability to this sickness. In other words, a far greater yin than everyday excessive intake of yin foods is the cause of this disease. Therefore, eat a yang diet: 2 teaspoons of gomasio at mealtime and another before bed.

Thrombosis:

Same as insomnia. Main food: special rice soup and buckwheat cream.

Yawning:

Signals serious illness. Follow the preliminary diet strictly. After a few days, yawning will disappear.

B. Eyes

Astigmatism:

Yin astigmatism prevents you from seeing horizontal lines clearly. The yang type prevents you from seeing vertical lines clearly. Both types can be cured by well-balanced (satvic) eating.

Blindness:

Caused by the mother's eating excess yin during pregnancy or nursing.

All "congenital" blindness can be cured by changing the mother's and baby's constitutions—up to the age of 8—by adhering to the preliminary diet or the special diet.

Cataracts:

Preliminary diet. Like diabetes, eat aduki beans and hokkaido pumpkin. Eat yang vegetables and grains and take 1-2 teaspoons of gomasio daily.

Color Blindness:

Again, there are two opposing types of color-blindness—yang (red) and yin (blue and green). Eat a well-balanced diet.

Conjunctivitis:
Preliminary diet and totally avoid all animal products including fish and dairy.

Eyelids—Inflamed or Running:
No special treatment or surgical operation is necessary. Simply follow the preliminary diet and avoid animal products. Your grain/vegetable ratio may be as great as is comfortable.

Farsightedness:
Caused by excess yang in the diet. Follow the preliminary diet, but use minimum salt and do not reduce liquid intake. (See illustration.)

Glaucoma:
Caused by too much yin foods, especially fats and alcoholic drinks. Observe preliminary diet. Drink as little as possible.

Retina—Detached or Bleeding:
This is a yin sickness, cured by several day's yang eating.

Nearsightedness:
Two types exist: yin and yang. Excess yin expands and elongates the globe of the eye so parallel rays are focused in front of the retina. Excess yang contracts the lens with the rays focused behind the retina. Balance the diet in either case or use yin or yang preparations as indicated by the case at hand. (See illustrations on the next page.)

C. Ears
Deafness and Dumbness:
Preliminary diet. In the case of a young baby, the mother should eat at least 70 percent grains. If the child is older, all members of his family should eat this way. Up to the age of 10, children may absolutely expect a cure.

EYE ILLUSTRATIONS

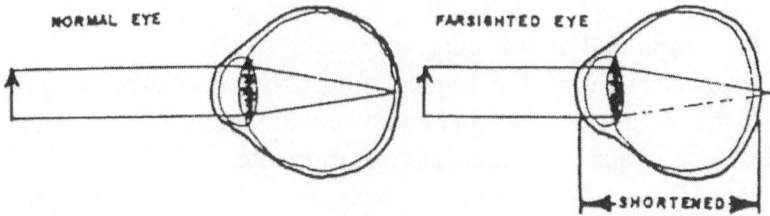

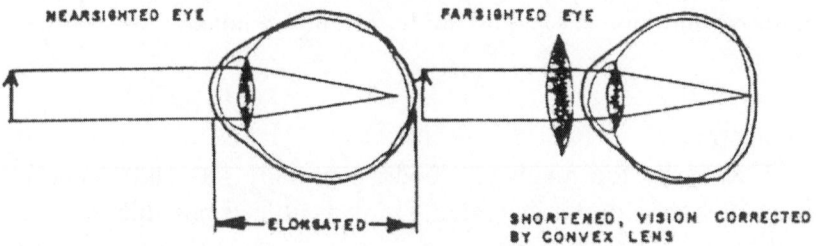

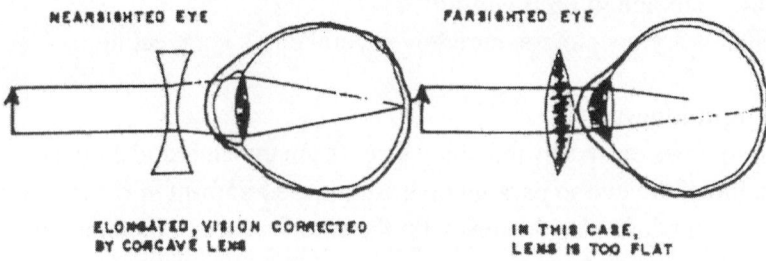

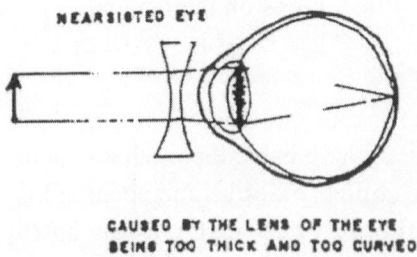

NORMAL EYE

FARSIGHTED EYE

SHORTENED

NEARSIGHTED EYE

ELONGATED

FARSIGHTED EYE

SHORTENED, VISION CORRECTED
BY CONVEX LENS

NEARSIGHTED EYE

ELONGATED, VISION CORRECTED
BY CONCAVE LENS

FARSIGHTED EYE

IN THIS CASE,
LENS IS TOO FLAT

NEARSIGHTED EYE

CAUSED BY THE LENS OF THE EYE
BEING TOO THICK AND TOO CURVED

Middle Ear Infections:

Preliminary diet and 1-2 teaspoons of gomasio daily. (See recipe 76.)

D. Nose

Nasal Mucus, Discharge, or Polyps (swelling or mucus membrane growths common in nostrils):

Several days to several weeks of the preliminary diet. Also, 1 teaspoon of gomasio at mealtime, lotus root fried in sesame oil, and lotus tea three times a day with no other liquids.

Sinus Troubles:

Same as Nasal Mucus, Discharge, or Polyps.

E. Mouth

Pyorrhea:

Completely cured by the preliminary diet. Add one-half teaspoon gomasio at mealtime and rub dentie into the gums three times a day.

Toothache and Tooth Decay:

If you follow the preliminary diet, you will never suffer from toothaches. Use sea salt or dentie daily as tooth powder. A bit of dentie mixed with water to form a paste rubbed into the gum around the painful tooth will relieve suffering.

F. Face

Eczema:

No animal products. The preliminary diet will heal any skin disorders or eruptions, from the simplest to the most painful with deep bleeding cracks like the bark of an oak. Apply Nukayu locally (see recipe 81). In severe cases, try the special diet.

Freckles and Irregular Pigmentation:

Caused by years of excessive yin or tamasic eating, that is, foods with a high potassium/sodium ratio and certain elements that neutralize sodium in the body. People who have eaten peppers, chilies, vinegar, and green beans for several years may develop whitish or blueish splotches or eventually albinoism. The only real cure is to avoid these foods (detachment from sensory pleasure and self-centeredness).

Neuralgia, Tension, and Facial Mannerisms (Tics):

Will disappear with simple good-eating. Use gomasio and ginger compress three times a day, 15-30 minutes each time.

Pimples:

Cut out sugar. Drink less liquids and avoid watery foods. No animal foods and no dairy for several weeks. Preliminary diet.

G. Throat

Adenoidal Growth:

Can be cured in several weeks with the preliminary diet. Use ginger compress three times a day. Parents whose child has these growths should make sure that their whole family eats very well. Otherwise, in the future, they will have low resistance and be accident prone. Their children will be especially vulnerable to tuberculosis, encephalitis, polio, or measles and will die young.

Asthma:

This so-called incurable disease is quite easily arrested by eating 70-90 percent grains. Basic elementary raja yoga. Asthmatics suffering even 20 years can be cured in several weeks. This reveals to you the basic superiority of food (the source of life) as medicine, the root of our existence and essence, our freedom (health), happiness (peace), and integrity (wholeness of being). Lotus root as a vegetable and a tea, and one-half teaspoon gomasio at mealtime. Ginger compresses and albi plasters in case of extreme suffering.

Coughing and Whooping Cough:

Same as asthma. If a nursing baby gets whooping cough, the

mother should eat the preliminary diet and take 3 teaspoons of lotus root juice two or three times a day. The cough will be relieved in less than an hour. Shots and other drugs given to the mother during pregnancy and nursing or given directly to the baby, even in minute doses, will hinder the development of his judgment. The baby is both physiologically and psychologically a reflection of his mother's condition.

H. Neck and Shoulders
Congestion:
If you have trouble turning your head 180 degrees from left to right or touching your right shoulder with your right ear and left with left, the blood flow around the neck and shoulders is blocked and may be a forewarning of apoplexy (paralysis due to brain hemorrhage or arterial blockage). Eat 70-90 percent grains right away and apply ginger compress and albi plaster four times a day.

I. Chest
Angina Pectoris: (Constricting chest pain radiating from the heart region to the left shoulder and down the arm, accompanied by cardiac oppression and apprehension of immediate death due to spasm in a major artery or to the presence, within the artery, of a blood-filled tumor. Also Angina Motoria, where the breast pang is comparatively slight with pallor, followed by the feet and hands turning blue and numb with cold):

Eat very well (preliminary diet), including 1-2 teaspoons gomasio a day and 1 teaspoon at bedtime. Ginger compress and albi plaster four times a day. Special whole rice cream.

Bone Decay—Ribs, Spinal Column, Hips:
Preliminary diet. Ginger compress and albi plaster four times a day. ½-1 teaspoon gomasio at mealtime.

Breast Cancer:
See stomach cancer and ulcers. Ginger compress followed by

albi plaster five times a day. ½-1 teaspoon gomasio at mealtime. Special diet.

Bronchitis:
Same as asthma. Whole rice soup or special rice cream. ½-1 teaspoon gomasio at mealtime. In extreme cases, ginger compresses and albi plasters.

Esophageal Cancer:
Ginger compresses and albi plasters. Whole rice soup or buckwheat cream with gomasio (½-1 teaspoon at mealtime). Special diet.

Gall Stones:
See kidney stones.

Heart Disease:
Preliminary diet. ½-1 teaspoon gomasio at meal time; 1 teaspoon before bed. Study chapter, "What is a Cardiac Condition?"

Liver Trouble (including jaundice and vomiting of bile):
Eat less and fewer rich foods (rich in caloric content, that is, oil and sugar). A month of partial fasting or the special diet for one week especially in the case of jaundice. Total fasting may be indicated. Ginger compress and albi plaster four times a day.

Lungs Inflamed or Pleurisy:
Same as nephritis (inflammation of the kidneys). Ginger compresses and albi plasters. Special whole rice cream.

Tuberculosis, Pulmonary:
See asthma.

J. Abdomen
Appendicitis:
Tofu or albi plaster four times a day. Whole rice cream with root

vegetables sautéed in sesame oil. In acute cases, 3 tablespoons of burdock juice. If burdock juice doesn't work, give 1 cup of chickweed juice.

Constipation:
Preliminary diet. Chick peas browned in sand (for even roasting) three times a day with tea or 1 cup cooked aduki beans, no salt.

Cysts (especially on reproductive organs):
Preliminary diet, strictly. Rub with ginger compresses then albi plasters. No operation or other treatment is necessary. If a child develops cysts, look to ineffective functioning of the internal organs (inability to transmute) in the parents, heart conditions, or other yin diseases caused by too much vitamin C, sugar, fruit, or raw vegetables.

Cystitis (bladder discharge):
Aduki soup—three bowls a day. Preliminary diet. Ginger compress three times a day.

Duodenal Ulcer:
Preliminary diet. 1-2 teaspoons gomasio a day and every hour a pinch very well-chewed. (See stomach ulcer).

Dysentery-amoebic or bacillic:
Preliminary diet. Take as much gomasio as possible. Ginger compresses or ginger hip baths are helpful.

Dyspepsia:
1-2 days fasting. Then whole rice soup or a cup of kuzu.

Gall Bladder Condition (with discharge of bile into blood stream or into stomach):
See liver trouble. ½-1 teaspoon gomasio at mealtime. Ginger compresses.

Gas:
Preliminary diet, strictly. Two ounces roasted chick peas with tea daily and as much gomasio as your system will tolerate.

Heartburn:
Gomasio. Preliminary diet or special diet for a shorter time.

Hemorrhoids:
If rectum is very inflamed, use ginger compresses or albi plasters. If a hemorrhoid is bleeding or very inflamed, chew on a piece of ginger (about thumb size). Do this only once. The ginger will taste really good at this time, though normally it tastes very hot and pungent. All pain and bleeding should stop. Strict adherence to the special diet.

Hernia:
Preliminary diet, strictly. In extreme cases, ginger compresses and albi plasters. 1-2 teaspoons gomasio at mealtime. A couple of pieces of shio kombu a day. Hernias in babies are caused by the mother's excessive yin eating.

Hiccups:
½-1 teaspoon gomasio a day. 1-2 bowls of syoban. Preliminary diet.

Indigestion:
Preliminary diet. Chew very well. ½-1 teaspoon gomasio at mealtime. Physical activity (cleaning, scrubbing, manual housework) at least 2-3 hours a day.

Kidneys (nephritis, tuberculosis, uremia):
Preliminary diet, strictly. Aduki beans and aduki soup, 2 cupfuls daily, lightly salted. Ginger compresses and albi plasters on kidneys. For uremia (excess urea or nitrogenous waste in blood) take radish drink No. 2 once a day for a maximum of 3 days. This drink may

also be used for swollen face and legs. (See Internal Treatment.)

Obesity:
Preliminary diet strictly. Three tablespoons sesame oil with sautéed vegetables daily. Two ounces raw daikon daily.

Ovaries Inflamed:
Preliminary diet. Ginger compress and albi plaster four times a day in severe cases. Chlorophyll hip baths (hibayu) 15 minutes before bed. (See External Treatment.)

Pancreas Trouble:
Preliminary diet. [Also millet. Chew very well.]

Stomach Cancer:
Preliminary or special diet. One-half teaspoon dentie swallowed in capsule or in a bit of bread, twice a day. Ginger compress and albi plaster five times a day. Buckwheat is good for cancer.

Stomach Cramps:
One teaspoon gomasio or a cup of very hot tamari bancha. Ginger compresses. (See Internal Treatment.)

Stomach-distended:
Whole rice well-boiled or fried. Chapati or crepes should form 70-80 percent of meals. Chew well. Ginger juice rub or compress three times a day.

Stomach Ulcer:
There is a distinguished sharp pain, usually after meals, often vomiting. There is often undigested food in the vomit. One may also vomit blood, which must be distinguished from the case of tuberculosis vomiting. This vomited blood usually comes out with foods and has dark-colored clots. Sometimes black tar-like stuff comes out in the stool. A large vomiting may cause severe weakness.

Treatment: When one vomits blood, give strong bancha tea with salt. Give ginger compress on abdomen and apply albi plaster after the ginger compress.

Diet: Preliminary diet with 1 teaspoon gomasio. Chew very well (100-200 times each mouthful). When there is no appetite or in severe cases, give brown rice soup and brown rice tea. After 4-5 weeks following the above diet, then gradually change to cooked grains, rice cream, miso soup, and soft vegetables without fibers.

Stomach—swollen:
Preliminary diet. ½-1 teaspoon gomasio at mealtime. No external treatment is necessary.

Stones (kidney, gall, etc.):
Preliminary diet, strictly. Avoid fruit and yin drinks. In case of pain, ginger compresses and albi plasters. Two teaspoons gomasio at meals for 3-4 days, then ½-1 teaspoon per meal.

Testicles—inflammation caused by gonorrhea or tuberculosis:
Preliminary diet. For pain, ginger compresses and albi plasters. No operation is necessary.

Uterus Diseases:
Preliminary diet. Chlorophyll hip baths once a day. For morning sickness, take an earthenware dish, heat it well, break it, and crush it into powder. Pour boiling bancha over the powder and cover. Before it cools, drink the top part—½ cup daily. Two teaspoons gomasio at mealtime. Similar treatment may be used for cancer of the uterus.

Vomiting (mucus discharge from stomach):
Take whole rice soup 3 days. Ginger compresses for pain.

K. Legs
Elephantiasis:
Preliminary diet, strictly. Absolutely no beans or peas except

adukis. Two teaspoons gomasio at mealtime. Daikon drink No. 2 once a day for 3 days only. Ginger compress twice a day. Albi plaster twice a day. Vegetables sautéed in 5 teaspoons sesame oil daily. Millet, whole wheat flour, buckwheat, oatmeal, rice, or barley, ½-1 cup daily. Two tablespoons raw daikon.

Flat Feet:

May be cured by changing the mother's diet. Flat feet may sometimes take on a new form, that of idiocy, imbecility, weakness, encephalitis, polio, tuberculosis, or—at the very least—prevent walking and running for any great distance.

Polio:

Preliminary diet. The mother who eats according to the Order of Nature will never see polio in her family. As much millet, buckwheat, and barley as possible. Three teaspoons gomasio daily. Whole wheat flakes and crackers. Whole rice, chick peas/lotus root, carrots, squash (especially the seeds), thistle root, dandelion, spinach, cress, wild vegetables like pigweed, and above all, hairy-rooted vegetables. Ginger compresses and albi plasters are indispensable. Imo plasters (this is natural potato-jinenjo plaster) are especially effective.

Polio can be cured in 1 or 2 weeks, if the patient is less than 12 or 13 years old; even cases of 10 years standing may be cured in a couple of months. In the United States, only one-third of polio victims are cured; the rest are paralyzed. Mortality rate due to polio is very high. Special diet for as long as 3 months may be necessary.

L. Whole Body

Allergies:

Preliminary diet will cure all allergies, incredible as it may seem.

Beriberi:

Whole rice, whole wheat, or buckwheat flour products should

constitute 80 percent of daily food, with 20 percent vegetables sautéed in sesame oil. Takuan and nuka pickles (a radish pickle—See *Chico-San Cookbook,* No. 107 and 108) to restore intestinal flora destroyed by extreme yin such as antibiotics or other drugs is good.

Colds and Flu:

No animal in its natural state catches cold. When man alone in the animal kingdom makes himself vulnerable to colds, he lowers himself physically, intellectually, and spiritually; he relinquishes his innate freedom. Goats thrive in harsh, biting, relentless winds; polar bears romp happily in icy waters. Suffering from the cold in a climate as warm as India's is indeed laughable. (Check your own condition against the seven criteria of health.) We are born to enjoy this world totally free, happy, and at one with life. Heat, cold, wind, suffering, and unhappiness hammer on the free man. If you are wiped-out by these forging blows, then you must be reborn. Start your life over by eating your earthly mother's food—70-90 percent grains. We are continually creating ourselves because we are the children [(▲) manifestation of the universe (▼), tao, infinite expansion], just as it is written in the *Vedas* and the *Bhagavad-Gita.*

Special whole rice soup, daikon drink No. 1 once. Suffering from a cold is the beginning of all unhappiness.

Diabetes:

The first postwar international conference of American specialists in diabetes declared that the insulin synthesized by Doctors Benting and Best was not only ineffective but also harmful. That was 25 years after its original synthesis. In its path lie thousands of victims' lives. The two Nobel Prize winners are no longer living— two criminals against the Order of Nature. This sickness—along with asthma, rheumatism, and polio—is one of the easiest to cure by practicing the macrobiotic way of eating. No matter how long you have been diabetic, a couple of weeks should bring relief. Aduki beans and hokkaido pumpkin. (Also see pancreas.)

Fatigue:
Bancha with gomasio or soy sauce.

Hydrophobia (rabies):
Preliminary diet broadly immunizes you against sudden suscep-
tibility to any virus. Daikon drink No. 2, rice cream and whole rice
soup; 2-3 teaspoons gomasio.

Leprosy:
There is no more effective medicine for leprosy than the way
of eating, simple living, raja yoga. Preliminary diet, very strictly.
Ginger compresses and albi plasters daily. ½-1 teaspoons gomasio
at meals.

Paralysis, Spasms, Parkinson's Disease:
Fasting for a couple of days or weeks. Eat only what is necessary
for your health. Preliminary diet.

Rheumatism:
Preliminary diet, strictly. Whole rice cream, gomasio. Ginger
compresses and albi plasters.

M. Cravings, Habits, and Addictions
Alcohol, Opium, Drugs:
Preliminary diet. Specific treatments are indicated by physical
symptoms.

N. Infections
Chicken Pox:
Whole rice cream with gomasio (1-3 teaspoons all at once,
wrapped in Nori or bread if preferred) and 3 tablespoons of wild
greens like watercress or dandelion, sautéed in sesame oil.

Cholera:
Whole rice cream and kuzu cream. Ginger compresses on the

stomach or a sitz bath with salt. If this doesn't stop the diarrhea, give a very warm, salty enema. Then follow with the preliminary diet.

Gastritis and Gastroenteritis:
See cholera.

Malaria:
Daikon drink No. 1. Preliminary diet. Take small amounts of gomasio between meals. Following the macrobiotic diet is perfect immunization. Today there are 100 million who suffer and 750 thousand who die from this sickness in India alone.

Measles:
Keep warm and drink special whole rice cream with kuzu. No yin preparations including daikon soup. The younger you catch measles, the more yang your constitution is. People over 10 with measles have a relatively tamasic or yin constitution.

Rat Bites:
Only very yin blood attracts rats (also mosquitoes, etc.). Eat only special whole rice cream. Albi plasters.

Scarlet Fever and Yellow Fever:
See malaria.

Small Pox:
Absolutely no liquids. Same as kidney conditions.

Typhoid Fever:
Same as dysentery, diarrhea, and malaria.

Diet After One Month on Preliminary

By Editor

The preliminary diet sometimes does not cure all of the sicknesses, even symptomatically, in a month's time. It takes more than one month to cure the symptoms even by good diet observation. Then, many wonder how to eat after one month because Ohsawa advises not to continue the preliminary diet for more than one month without consulting someone who knows better. Yet, he doesn't tell how to eat or what to eat after the preliminary diet. Therefore, we feel it is better that we give some idea on how to continue the macrobiotic diet after the preliminary diet.

The diet following the preliminary diet is not much different from the preliminary one. The main difference between the two is mostly in the quantity of grains eaten. In the preliminary diet, Ohsawa recommends 70-90 percent grains. However, for most Americans, this will be too strict and inevitably cause a strong craving for meats, chicken, cheese, or sweets. Therefore, we recommend not to continue with 70-90 percent grains for more than one month. Instead, broaden the diet as explained in *Macrobiotics: An Invitation to Health and Happiness* (see chart on next page).

Vegetables:

Any except tomatoes, potatoes, and eggplant because these are too yin for the sick. Can be sautéed, pressure cooked, baked, fried. However, very yang persons or some whose symptoms are

171

very yang may eat these excluded vegetables in-season if one craves these foods. If you crave some foods, don't restrict too hard, but rather eat them. Otherwise, the craving may become bigger and bigger and finally explode to a huge bingeing. Also, too rigid restriction may cause psychological, emotional rigidity, which disturbs smooth energy flow in the body. As a result, symptoms of depression, no energy, sluggishness, etc. appear. Therefore, such rigid restriction may be worse than eating these foods.

Beans:

All beans, especially aduki beans, black beans, chick peas, and lentils.

Seaweeds:

Nori, kombu, wakame, hiziki, etc. See *Do of Cooking, Vol. 2.*

Salt:

The amount of salt used in cooking is one of the most critical techniques in macrobiotics. One who has eaten much animal foods may not do well eating much salty foods. However, not enough salt may cause sluggishness. Therefore, everyone should find the amount of salt that brings him to his best condition. If someone cooks for you, you may not be able to choose the amount of salt in the foods you eat. In such cases, don't eat too much cooked vegetables or salt pickles because they contain a lot of salt by cooking. In conclusion, if one works hard, he can take more salt than one who doesn't work so much physically.

This is true also for one person who can take more salt when he is working hard than when he does not.

Also, salty foods are tasty and stimulate the stomach, and we tend to overeat. As a result, we become too salty (yang—muscle constriction, rigidity, anger). The remedy for this is only to work hard. If you eat too much, then you better work hard. This burns up extra foods so that there is no extra energy in the body, which often causes nervousness, irritation, sluggishness, and worry.

Activity:

If you want to cure quickly, keep busy and work hard, even when you are weak. For some people, skipping one meal, or two meals even, will help to maintain a good state of mind and physical condition. This is recommended for people having trouble with overeating. If you eat only once or twice a day you can eat a larger amount each time. This often helps to keep the total daily intake lower.

Fish:

Fish flakes and/or chuba iriko (small whole fish) can be used in soup or other cooking on a daily basis, if desired. When using them, you will need considerably less or no salt. In hot weather, you can completely eliminate fish in most cases. Recipes for some fish will be in the following chapter.

Animal Foods:

Animal foods are better avoided even after the preliminary diet because they cause an acidic condition of the blood, are too yang for most Americans, and are contaminated with many chemicals, etc. If one craves animal foods, he is discharging the excess protein that has accumulated for many years of a meat diet. In such cases, better to eat vegetable protein foods such as natto (fermented soybeans), tofu (soybean curd), any beans, miso soup, etc.

Sweets:

For the first few days, weeks, or even years of observing the macrobiotic diet, it may be difficult to eliminate the craving of sweets. For this, you'd better learn how to make nice macrobiotic desserts made of sweet rice, aduki beans, squash, amasake (see *Do of Cooking Vol. 4*), chestnuts, berries, apples, etc., especially for the diabetic. In any case, for the sick, better avoid honey, sugar, and excess of fruits. However, this again must be balanced with your craving.

Pressed Salads and Pickles:

Many vegetables can be pressed and pickled. These salads and

	Winter Cold Climate	Fall/Spring Temp. Climate	Summer Hot Climate
Grains	70-90%	50-70%	30-60%
Vegetables	10-20	30-50	40-70
which includes:			
Beans	5-10	5-12	10-15
Seaweed	5-10	5-12	10-15
Pressed Salad	0-10	5-12	8-15
Fish	10	5	2

pickles are very important foods and are best served at every meal, because they—especially rice or wheat bran pickles—will help to build lactobacilli in the intestines, which in turn can produce several B vitamins. Vitamin B helps the metabolism of glucose. In other words, without vitamin B, one will not produce enough energy even though he may have enough glucose in his system. In many cases, the craving for sugar (sweets) is the result of a lack of vitamin B. (See *Do of Cooking, Vol. 1 and 3* for salad and pickle recipes.)

Overeating:

Overeating is the main problem among long-time macrobiotics. After several years of macrobiotic eating, one loses the desire to eat meat and sugar. His diet is quite stable. The only trouble is he has too strong an appetite. The macrobiotic diet is too delicious and health-making. Ohsawa wrote about his own difficulties to overcome over-eating in his Japanese book long ago. He concluded the following methods to overcome the trouble:

1. Sleep early and get up early because early morning is very yin, which controls yang greediness.

2. Chew well. If we chew 100 times or more each mouthful of food we eat, we will be tired from eating.

3. Skip breakfast or lunch or both. Choose whichever is best suited to you.

4. Share foods with others. If you have a quart of ice cream, don't eat by yourself but make a party so that your portion of eating is small. If you crave a honey cake, don't buy it for you only, but buy for friends too. This giving and sharing mentality has a great power that can dominate the egoistic, self-centered cravings. After eating a little bit of sweets, or anything you want, your ego desire is satisfied, and you will be quite contented. Otherwise, you may be ashamed from your greediness, and sinful feelings remain after eating. Often, bingeing itself is not harmful, but the psychological and emotional resentment of oneself causes much more harm.

In other words, the giving or sharing mentality is more important than what you eat in some cases, because the state of emotions influences the condition of organs, functions of the nervous system, and the secretion of hormones.

In macrobiotics, someone tends to think from the standpoint of nutrition or physical health or yin and yang of foods. And someone else tends to think from the standpoint of the spiritual or mental aspect. However, we should look at macrobiotics from both sides, because they are one. Therefore, one who tends to think materialistically, better try to be more spiritual. And one who tends to think spiritually or psychologically, better try to be more materialistic and practical.

In this book, therefore, we present macrobiotic medicine in both ways. The first half of the book is the practical and materialistic approach of macrobiotic medicine, and the second half is the spiritual approach.

Hand Healing
By Lima Ohsawa

Everyone has the ability to heal with his hands. By instinct, one places his hand over the painful area when hurt. Our hands have energy vibrations; they can cure many troubles. Perhaps this is symptomatic, but no drugs or equipment are necessary so one can utilize hand healing at any time or place. A good diet is, of course, the basis of health, cleaning up sickness from the inside. But, hand healing still has a place in obtaining good health. With practice, one can gain power, and the aptitude will increase quickly. To practice once or twice is not enough, so please try many times with many friends. A dog or other animal licks a wound to aid the healing process, and a mother kisses her child's sore. Healing with the hands is a similar process.

Techniques for Specific Healing

Common Cold:

A cold is almost always from too much eating. Place your thumb at the central point, at the base of the ribs. Use just a light touch, pressure is not necessary. With practice one will be able to feel a sharp pain in his hand when the patient has a serious disease. Remove the hand after 15 minutes.

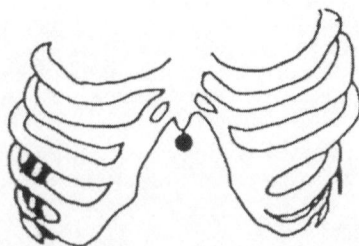

Headache or Fever:

Place hand on the forehead for 20-30 minutes. When there is a fever, much sweat will come off of the forehead; at this point, remove hand quickly. If there is no sweating, the hand can remain for 1-2 hours, but when sweat comes the fever will have broken and will be going down. A patient will be healed much more quickly when he is grateful.

Liver:

The liver is connected with the eyes, so by placing the hands over the eyes, pain in the liver may be relieved.

Spleen:

Same as the liver, place hands over the eyes. This is also effective for ear trouble as the ear and spleen have a connection. The spleen also affects the nose and is sometimes the cause of a fatigued condition. Treat for 20 minutes.

Small Intestine:

Place hand over the small intestine. In children, pain will go quickly, and color should return to the cheeks.

Female Troubles:

Place hand over the abdomen. If there are uterus problems, one will often have nose trouble so the hand can be placed on the nose. After 1 hour, there should be no more pain from cramps.

Kidney Troubles:

The kidneys are also connected with nose troubles. Place hand under the arch of the back for 20 minutes. All skin problems are because of poor kidneys.

Heart Troubles:

Place hand over the left side of the chest. If the patient has serious heart problems, the hand should be placed very slowly over the heart so that the patient will not have any pain. The magnetism will work as the hand approaches, contracting the body. For heart troubles, one can firmly squeeze the end of the little finger; this will improve circulation to the heart. Sometimes heart trouble is due to poor circulation.

Lung Troubles:

Place hands directly over the lungs.

Rheumatism, Arthritis, Car Accident:

Place hand directly over painful area.

Ear Troubles:

If there is pain, move hand slowly towards the ear. This is a very sensitive area, and the magnetism will work. When the hand is placed over the ear, the middle finger may be inserted.

Toothache:

Apply dentie over painful area, place fingers under jawbone along chin, and push gently.

Hemorrhoids:

Place the middle finger at the anus and the thumb forward toward the spine. Sometimes the intestines will be pushed out. At this time, a gentle massage maybe given, and they should move back. Treat for 20 minutes.

When hand healing is practiced, the patient should wear one layer of cotton clothing; too much clothing will weaken the effects. One can do hand healing alone or with the aid of another person. The right hand is almost always used, but the left or both hands may also be used.

Treatment for the Whole Body

With the patient lying on his stomach, place your left hand over your right hand at the top of the spine, giving pressure with the left hand. Quickly move the hands to the base of the spine, concentrating pressure with the fingers. Repeat this 30 times; it is good for the nervous system. Next, brush hands from the spine towards the sides along the ribs; also, quickly brush hands from the shoulder towards the elbow.

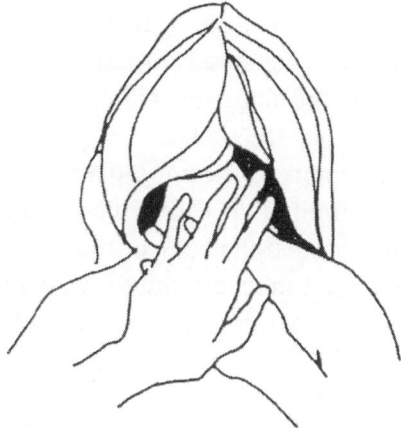

Push the left hip (with your hand under the buttocks) toward the right shoulder, and the right hip toward the left shoulder.

Lift the leg, touching the heel to the buttocks, release, and let it drop to the floor. Do this several times with each leg separately and then with both legs together.

Lift each leg, bending at the knee, and with the sole of the foot facing up; pound the bottom of the foot with your fist. Use long, rhythmic strokes. As the feet carry all the body weight, this will relax the entire body.

Pull the toes one by one, and, with the side of the hand, brush the toes back and forth 10 or 20 times.

With the patient sitting in a folded leg position and breathing through the nose, place your thumbs at the center base of the skull and press

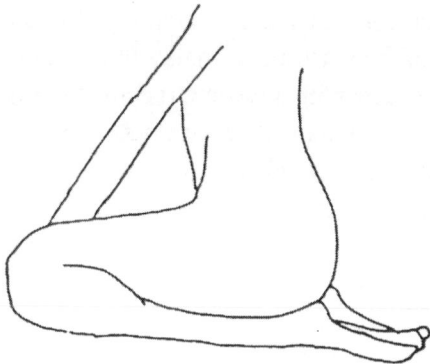

toward the forehead.

With the index finger, apply pressure on the inside of the eye socket. This is good for fatigue or sleepiness. For fatigue, one can also moisten the fingertip with saliva and brush gently along the eyelids.

To improve memory, place the little fingers in front of the ears and cup the rest of the fingers around the back of the head. This position should be maintained for 5 minutes: pull forward quickly when removing hands.

Every morning upon waking, sit with your heels under buttocks, knees one fist apart, and hands in a praying posture with tops of fingers level with your nose. Maintain this posture for 5 minutes, clearing the mind of all thoughts. If you feel pain in the legs, move to another position. Breathe deeply and evenly while in this posture. After 5 minutes of sitting, push the air from your throat, making a low vibrating noise. This routine will increase your healing powers. If you feel a sensation in the hands when they are folded, then the powers are working.

Sensitivity should be developed in the hands so that body temperatures can be felt. The warmest area on the patient's body is the weakest one.

When one gives a massage or does hand healing, the healer's body gives energy to the patient. There is also a transference of bad energy from the patient to the healer. Energy may be replenished with fresh air and by slapping the hands together with long strokes in the prayer formation, do this about five times. Vigorously shaking the hands with a loose wrist also eliminates accumulated energy.

If one does not eat animal food hand, healing powers will come much more quickly.

In making rice balls, one should form the rice with the hands. By doing this, the rice will absorb good energy and become very delicious.

Jesus used hand healing. With exercise, good food, and daily practice we can develop strong hand healing powers.

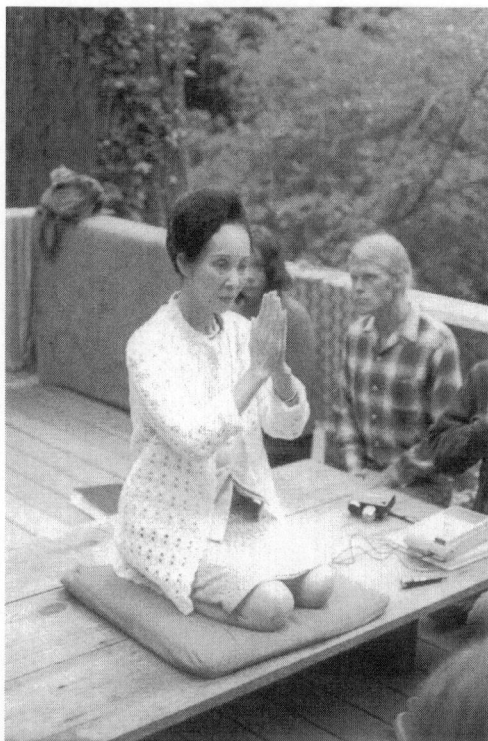

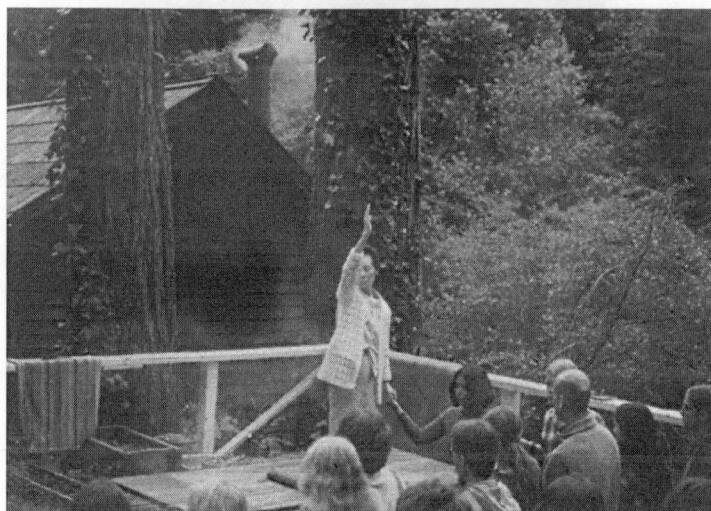

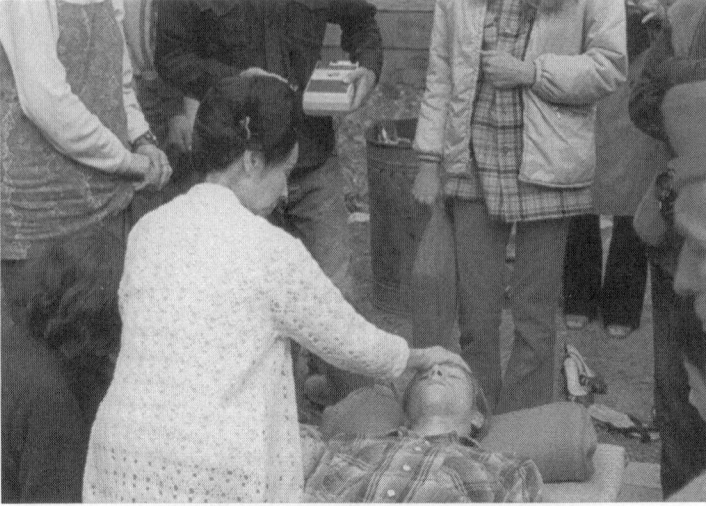

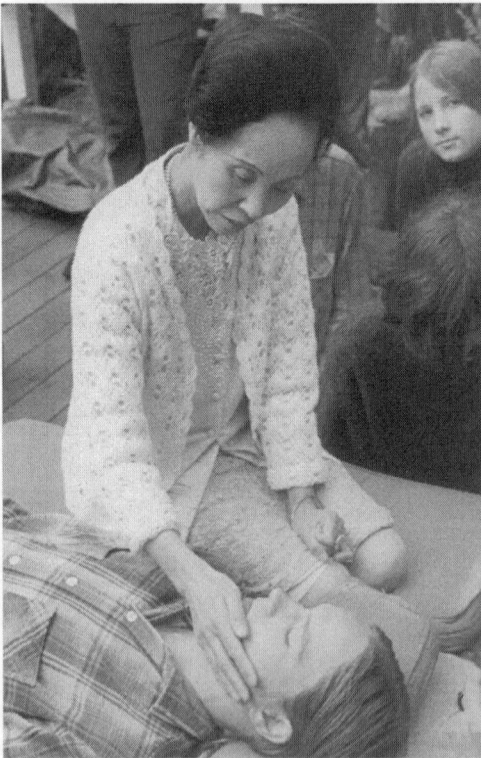

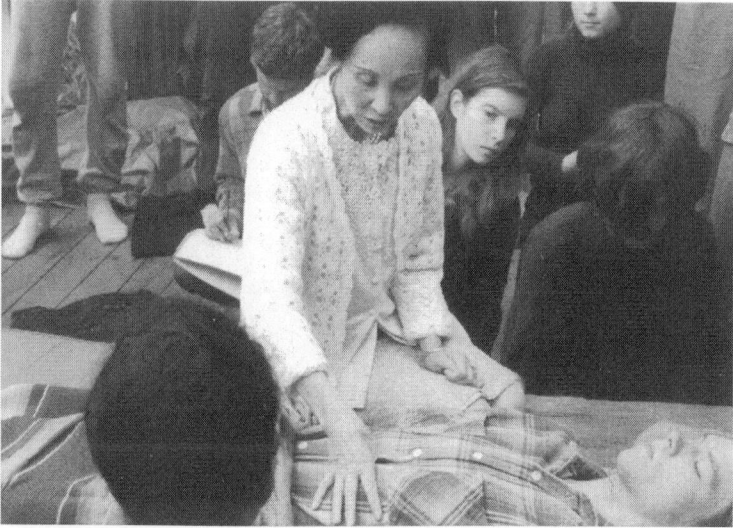

Massage
By Lima Ohsawa

There are points for the entire nervous system along the spine, so massaging the spine is very important. Always examine the spine by bending the patient forward from a sitting position. If the spine is curved towards one side, it is not good.

To massage, use the flat pad of the thumb and, with a spirallic motion, press ½ inch each side of each vertebra from neck to tail. Keep the thumb in a straight line with the arm for the best pressure. A knot or firm area on the back indicates pain. Massage down the spine three times then cross the thumbs, pressing down each side three more times. Finally, inhale and quickly but firmly push with the thumbs all the way down the sides of the spine. Always try to breathe with the patient.

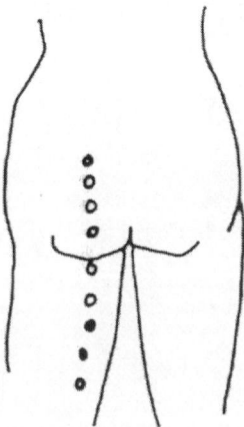

Gently push from the back out to the shoulders. Press the important points down the center of the buttocks and all along the back of the legs on the gall bladder meridian. (See figure to left.)

Massage the bottom of the heel with a cupped hand in a spiral motion. Massage the center arch area (kidney point). Do each of these three times for excellent relief of fatigue from walking. Squeeze all along each toe three or more times. Rotate the ankle in both directions.

184

Touch the heel to the buttocks. If the patient is not loose-jointed, do this slowly, and do each leg separately, then both together.

The belly button is the center of the abdominal area. With the flat of the entire hand gently massage around belly button in a clockwise direction (see below). The next movement should be with the palm of both hands; push hands across the stomach and pull back with stress on the fingers. Do this for 5 minutes to relieve constipation.

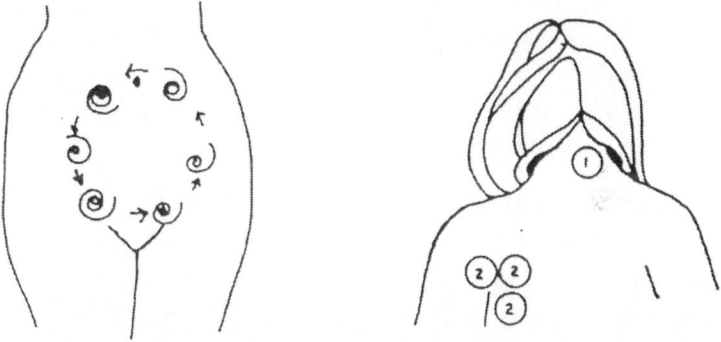

Brush firmly with thumbs down the spine. With palms, brush from the spine out along the ribs. Massage the area around the armpit and shoulder blade (No. 2 above right).

Massage up and down arms and along hand meridians.

With palms flat, move in an infinity pattern over kidneys. There is no need for strong pressure; movement creates warmth.

Massage buttocks, press with thumbs the points on the lower buttocks (right, No. 1). Pressure should be firm and direction towards shoulders.

Press with thumbs along the muscle lines on the back of the legs (right, No. 2). The hand should be clenched. With a quick, short, back and forth motion move

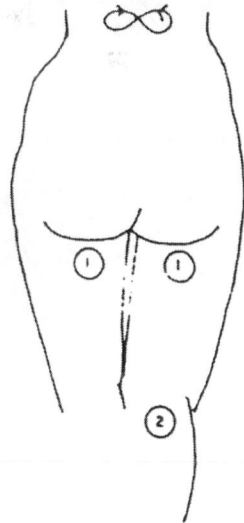

down the legs from thigh to ankle.

Massage the leg in bent position (below right), then quickly pull the foot down. Do this for both legs.

Massage the heel with a cupped palm, move the heel gently, as much as possible.

If the liver is bad, pay special attention to the points along the outside edge of the foot.

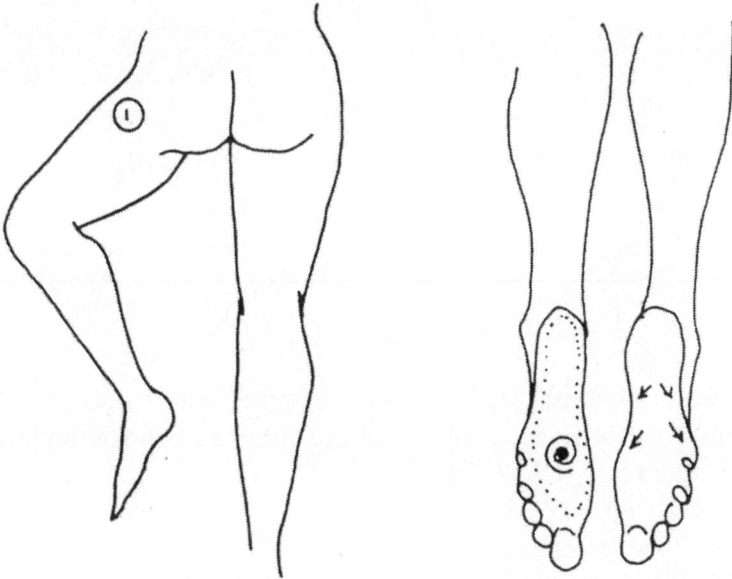

For the stomach, massage the point just between the ball and arch of each foot (see above, left foot). With thumbs, press outward down feet (see above, right foot).

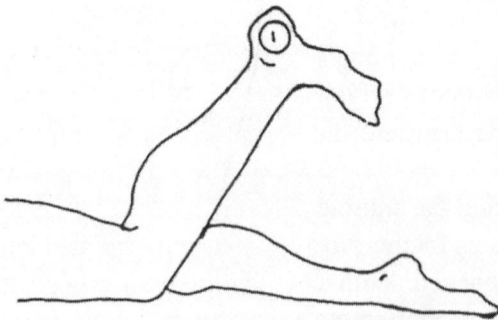

With leg bent, pound the sole of the foot (left, No. 1).

With thumb press the intestine points

from neck to outside shoulders. This may be repeated several times. There are very important points along the outside of the shoulder blades. Using entire hands, brush from the spine out to the sides.

Place one hand on the forehead and the other at the back of the skull. Then massage the scalp. Pound the scalp with your fingertips; be careful if you have long nails. With one hand on top of the head, push upwards at the lower central skull. Gently chop along the outside of the neck with your hand. By using the open fingers on the scalp, a yin/yang polarity is created. This helps to contract the mind. Massage with thumbs in a spiral motion at the base of the skull, just behind the ears (see fig. top left of next page, No. 1).

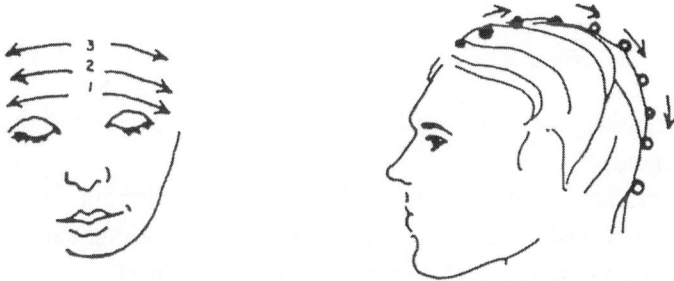

When the patient is lying on his back, massage with thumbs just above the eyes. Press in an outward direction to the temples—move up to the hairline (fig. above left).

Press with thumbs along the center of the scalp, from the hairline back towards the neck. Using both hands with the fingers loose, chop on scalp, sides first, then center (fig. above right).

Press the large intestine points on the shoulders with thumbs (fig. top left of next page, No. 2). Press the points just below the collarbone, from the neck going out toward the shoulders. Massage along the upper arm with the entire hand; skip the elbow, massage to the wrist. Lock fingers around hand, exposing patient's palm. Massage with thumbs, especially on intestine point (fig. top right of next page, No. 1) and liver point (same fig., No. 2). Hold the elbow and twist the lower arm at the elbow by moving the hand back and forth. Hold

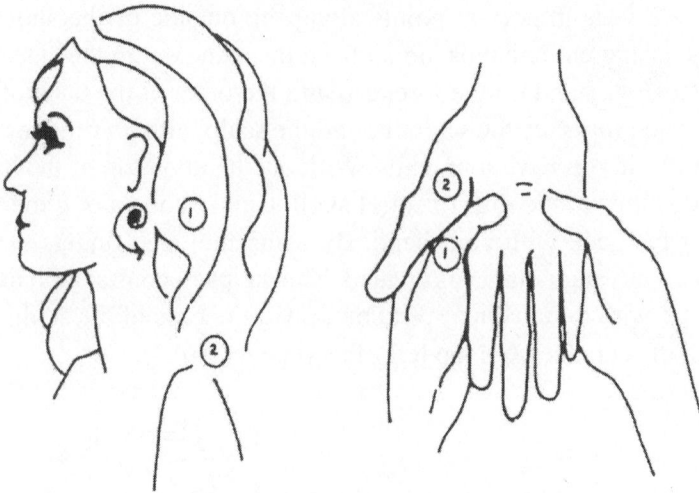

the patient's palm with your fingers touching his and stroke the back of his hand.

With thumbs, press along both sides of the shinbone. This is for both the stomach and kidney meridians. Massage along each side of the leg, stressing important points from thigh to ankle.

Twist foot at ankle in a clockwise and counterclockwise motion. Bend the foot forward and backward. When the foot is pushed forward (fig. right, No. 1), it helps restore circulation. It is especially good to massage the feet when one is faint as this is usually due to poor blood circulation. Hold the leg firm and twist feet out towards the sides.

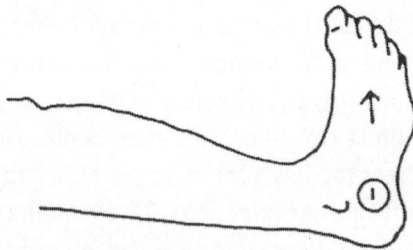

With both palms, press around the belly button and over the entire abdomen. Place hands under the small of the back in the kidney area; lift and release quickly several times.

Part 3

Cure the Man

When Will You Be Cured?

A medical doctor wrote me a criticism after the summer camp:

"Regarding any criticism of yourself, professor, we are all trying our best to learn of oriental philosophy and medicine. Whatever understanding or use we can and will make of your teachings, it must be realized that this will occur within the occidental culture we live in; therefore, we must be dependent on criteria that are compatible with our circumstances. When we say a patient is completely cured, their circumstances of cure must be such that any physician would examine the patient and accept them as being in good health, not just mentally at peace and happy, but still evidencing on physical examination or lab examination the same findings that might have been originally present. It does not suffice to say that our method and techniques of examination are inadequate and inaccurate. Whatever errors they represent are constant and relative. I would like to see you more willing to interpret your opinions in terms that would satisfy our occidental culture."

When will you be cured? "You will be cured in ten days to two months." I often answer your question so. And yet you do not find yourself cured within that period. Why? I have stated repeatedly that macrobiotics cures all diseases within ten days, that it changes the body's orientation toward health, away from disease, which teaches that disease is the exact barometer of our mistakes, or our abuse, of our ignorance of the Order of the Universe. It is therefore said that there can be no cure unless we recognize our own faults, our own ignorance, and, above all, the Order of the Universe, the key to our health, freedom, and our acknowledgement of perfect justice. But... what is justice? Everyone thinks he knows, but in reality...

According to Oriental philosophy, justice is absolute, infinite, eternal, and universal. A larger concept, by far, than that of Western justice. (See an American dictionary or the *Encyclopedia Brittanica* for the definition of justice.) The commonly understood meaning of justice is relative, personal, finite, and conditional. Democratic justice as defined by John Locke is known only by the majority. In actuality, there is no single concept in Western thought that is the equivalent of this concept.

Justice is another name for happiness that is infinite and eternal: A macrobiotic individual is a student of the way to such infinite happiness. The Unique Principle or, in other words, life itself, is the only teacher of this all-embracing justice.

Most of you look for a rapid cure and make large statements about your willingness to pay any price to achieve it. Still, you only attempt to understand basic Yin/Yang functioning where it concerns your immediate diet. Worse yet, you allow others to tell you what to eat. You abandon all pursuit of the Unique Principle as soon as your physical difficulties have disappeared. In short, the patient is never willing to pay the true price.

Two persons come to mind, both of whom were not cured by macrobiotics. Each had been crippled for a long time previously. Neither could understand that disease cannot leave the patient until he discovers and acknowledges his own mistakes. So many individuals are relieved of their anxieties and suffering by following the macrobiotic diet, yet become ill again because they do not probe ever deeper into the Unique Principle, the Law of Life.

I have understood, once and for all, that one must not cure anyone. Everyone must do it for himself, by himself. If your wish is to gain a reputation, to have a good income, to enjoy a sentimental self-esteem, you can, of course, make a career of taking care of people.

When will you be cured? In ten days, most assuredly, if you sincerely admit to yourself your own mistakes. The kind of disease makes no difference, since all diseases are a variation of man's loss of balance—biological, psychological or spiritual. If you are not cured in ten days or two months, you have no right to criticize my teaching. You have only to regret your own poor understanding of infinite and absolute justice.

Curing the Man

Macrobiotic practice can cure disease symptoms easily. The difficulty lies in curing the patient. He must learn how to unfetter himself, cast off his shackles, and walk upright, unafraid, a natural man, a free man. But learning to be free requires the total involvement of heart, imagination, faith, and will.

The technique to cure sickness is called medicine. To cure, one must know the cause of sickness. However, modern medicine does not know the cause. What modern medicine calls cause is merely symptoms or the results of sickness. The reason modern medicine cannot cure so many diseases is in the fact that it does not know the cause of disease.

Then what is the cause of disease?

In my opinion, the cause of disease is in the condition in which one's Supreme Judgment is clouded or eclipsed. All animals other than man have the lower judgment only, which is the first, second, and third stages of judgment; they are lacking the fourth, fifth and sixth stage of judgment. Therefore, they reveal the Supreme Judgment more easily than man. In the case of man, contrary to animals, having the fourth through sixth stages of judgment, the Supreme Judgment is eclipsed. Question: Why do the fourth, fifth, and sixth stages of judgment eclipse the Supreme Judgment?

Judgment is a compass of life giving us directions and decisions in our travels through life. One who has a wrong judgment goes a wrong direction, and the result is unhappiness or sickness. Sickness is the first warning that we have a wrong judgment. A healthy person never is unhappy. If so, his health is only physical, not total and real health; or his health is given from parents or others.

For example, however we analyze a picture by its amount, quality, and price of color used, we never improve the picture. The skill of the painter must be improved. For that, his thinking, idea, or concept of life must be improved. Modern medicine tries to cure sickness by analyzing the color. It is forgetting the painter completely who uses the color and designs the picture.

Most medicines are aiming at curing the symptoms. When it realizes that the symptomatic cure is useless or endless or dangerous, it turns to other ways. One of them is psychic, psychological, religious healing, and the other one is social and preventive medicine. However, any one of these has a tendency of symptomatic cure. Macrobiotic medicine aims at curing man, and not the sickness only, because man is the producer of sickness. Without curing man, no sickness is cured.

Western medicine must develop to a preventive medicine. The preventive medicine must develop to the way of health— Macrobiotics. The way of health must reach to the way of living. The principle of such a way of living must be simple and universal. Such principle should not be a difficult and sophisticated concept but must be an easy and practical one, which can be applied by anyone in daily life.

Mastering macrobiotic medicine means to become a man who devotes himself in search of infinite freedom, eternal happiness, and absolute justice, and to be a man who doesn't worry about money, power, knowledge, status, and fame. However you are skillful in any technique, you will be far from the real freedom, happiness, and justice if your aim is making money, status, or fame, etc. This is true in the case of medicine; the more the medicine becomes expensive, the more it becomes unjust, unfree, and unhappy. Air cooled by an air-conditioner is more expensive than air in the woods and is harmful to us. Sunlight is cheaper and healthier than any artificial light or radiation. Water from mountain streams without pollution is much cheaper and more health-giving than soda, orange juice (factory made), beer, and even drugs.

All plants grow by only sunshine, air, and water. And they are beautiful, strong, and gentle. Animals are the same. The Angora rabbit of Peru has immunity to all bacterial diseases. This finding made this animal an important animal in medical study. It lives in the high mountains of Peru where sunlight is weak and air is thin. The secret of immunity is he doesn't drink much. He drinks only for necessity. Excess water makes blood thin, which in turn weakens the immunity power and also thins out nutrition. As a result, it weakens the heart and kidneys. In short, excessive and greedy eating and drinking is the cause of all sicknesses. True medicine must be cheap and can be acquired in any place and any time.

Lao-tse said, "Winning without weapon is the real winning." Macrobiotic medicine is a medicine without weapons such as knives, needles, drugs and chemicals, and radiation.

Macrobiotic medicine is a teaching of awareness of the reality or the Order of Nature through sickness. In this sense, macrobiotic medicine is more religious than modern religions. In fact, macrobiotic people acquire the real religion, and not superstitions. In other words, when you realize that you are the cause of the sickness and sickness is the benefactor of your life, when you like everyone, when you reach the mentality of Will Rogers who said, "I never met a man I didn't like," when you appreciate anything including sickness, misfortune, and difficulties, then you graduate from macrobiotic medicine. To reach this state of mind, my practical method is the following:

Live with whole grains and vegetables using a bit of salt and oil and traditional condiments.

Chew 50 times or more each mouthful of food.

Drink as little as possible.

Work hard physically.

After three years of observing the above diet and the way of living, you can establish health. After that, teach Macrobiotics to others for seven years. Then, you devote yourself to whatever you want most in your life.

The Education of the Will

Translated by Fred Pulver from *YIN/YANG,*
French macrobiotic magazine, July-August, 1970, No. 107

Education—East and West

Modern Western education is scientific. Its ideal is the extension of understanding through data derived from the senses—second level judgment. This education has become professional and conformist technique.

The result of modern education is apparent in the behavior of 180 million people who populate the world. Our nation, for example, continues aerial bombardment 50 or 60 times a day, throws atrocious poisoned gas, uses modern chemical weapons daily that are the most murderous ever used up to the present day, and spends more than 10 million dollars a day on this warfare.

Thus it comes that hundreds of Vietcong are killed each day. They live only on whole brown rice, and own almost no weapons; they as well as hundreds of innocent, barefoot, wretched, pacifistic women and children die each day, victims of war, in this distant little country more than 10,000 kilometers from its aggressor.

In the beginning of the 19th century, Western education was founded on the idea that science creates superior conditions for human life. The great dream of science is that one day what is regarded as the greatest of all calamities, poverty, will be banished from the earth (read, *Matter* by Dr. Lapp).

Far Eastern education, which originated 5,000 years ago, was completely opposite from Western education. It taught that one should enjoy poverty and consider it a blessing. That one should regard difficulties and suffering with gratitude, as a help or guide—that a simple roof sufficed for shelter and that a handful of rice and a few vegetables were sufficient as food.

It taught that one should consider cold and heat as teachers that fortify, rather than treat them as enemies—that it is not necessary to kill animals, and even less necessary to kill bacteria. It also taught that one should adapt himself to everything and everyone, that one should treat others like a spring breeze while strengthening himself with the autumn frosts—that one should pardon others, respect others, and love everyone in the conviction that all is given inexhaustibly. That one should not hesitate to give his life for others. That one should devote himself to the search for truth; that is, the Unique Principle and practice in daily life, Peace, Purity, and respect of macrobiotics.

Education in the Far East was profoundly spiritual and taught that adaptation to nature is the way to arrive at Supreme Judgment. Later this was degraded by conformist and conceptual educators, who advocated a system that pretended to teach seeds and buds how to immediately become fruits and flowers. This new education produced a nationalistic robot-like people, obedient imitators, without the spirit of independence. It taught the youth of humanity to imitate the ideals and methods of the sages, which is impossible even for adults.

That's why, since the arrival of the seductive Western civilization, people immediately became slaves, not only materially but also spiritually. Thus, it created a colonized people.

For the past 100 years, Japan has accepted Western education with enthusiasm, and has put all its energy into becoming an imitator of Western civilization. This has led to the total defeat of Japan without precedent in the history of humanity. In the schools of America, the world's biggest stronghold of Western civilization, as well as in the Japan of today, one sees an extraordinary rise of criminality, mental sickness, allergies, heart diseases, cancer, iatrogenic diseases (diseases caused by drugs and medicines), the loss of the critical spirit, the inability to think, and the increase in retardation and use-lessness in children.

Thus, Far Eastern education, like that of the West, has made the Earth into a big spaceship in the form of a sphere, which flies at 10,000 km/hr carrying 3 billion individuals toward the depths of unhappiness, slavery, war, disease, suffering, and uncertainty. From this comes the necessity of discovering a new method of physiological and biological education.

The Fundamental Base of All Education

At 17, I was struck with tuberculosis, and my condition was so serious I was abandoned by modern medicine. I saved myself at the gates of death by the macrobiotic method, 5,000 years old. I would like to communicate to everyone the joy I feel I have arrived finally at 74 years of age, at the end of my work which, for 54 years, since I was 20 years old, has been to diffuse this method to the entire world. This has been a self-education as well as an education of the public at the same time.

Far Eastern medicine, originating 5,000 years ago, was not a medicine of symptoms, but a fundamental method of cure that is based on natural causes. This is why it was also a method of health, longevity, and happiness. It was not concerned with the disappearance of symptoms, but it was an educative medicine, which had as its end the development of man's judgment. This is revealed in the original theory of education of the old Chinese medicine, in the three great imperial disciplines of Japan, in the Code of Manu, in Ayurvedic medicine, in the alimentary disciplines of all the great religions of humanity, such as Buddhism, Jainism, Christianity, etc.

The five great religions of humanity were born in the East. They are the guiding fundamental conditions, the synthesis of theory and practice, the testimonial by its own life, of the monism that permits the establishment of a world of Peace, to realize the happy life that humanity desires. That is why it is quite evident that humanity must include the method of health, physiology, pathology, and medicine. But this understanding has grown dim over thousands of years, until it has been eclipsed finally and has disappeared before the importation of dualistic, materialistic, atomic, technical, modern civilization, whose judgment is based on brilliant and seductive appearances.

The primordial problem for man is the establishment of health. This is why we must give the greatest emphasis to the education of health and hygiene. All living creatures know how to control their own health except for man. Western medicine attaches all importance to the disappearance of symptoms. It does not search for the cause, and never tries to build up the source of vitality. Consequently, it has become a simple specialized technique; it has fallen into mere formality, and the educative spirit has completely disappeared. That is why modern medicine vegetates in an impasse, in spite of formidable technical progress. If, in days of old, one believed in this omnipotent medicine, which today is represented by the A.M.A., the dictator of America that even President Kennedy could not control, one must recognize its total defeat before these four sicknesses: cancer, heart diseases, mental illness, and allergic conditions, which are the cause of 70-80 percent of all deaths in America.

But the reality is worse, for not only are doctors incapable of curing these four great sicknesses, they can only postpone the death of men who suffer from general sicknesses and maintain them as patients, just as they cannot cure the common cold or rheumatism, or diabetes, or eczema, or any other chronic disease. As Claude Bernard said, "The true medicine does not yet exist," or as Bergson said, "The greatest fault of science is the ignorance of life." Dr. Rene Allendy also declared, "Pasteur, whose glory exceeds Napoleon's, has in reality weakened humanity, by destroying the system of natural selection, and blemished the history of French medicine and France."

In the Far East, ancient education was before all else a way of independence, the study of self, physiologically and biologically, and its goal was to follow a free and peaceful way through establishment of health by oneself, for oneself, and under one's control. The Orientals made a single way of medicine and education.

Thanks to the death of three of my nearest family members, since I was 10 years old, I vowed to discover the true cause of this absurd unhappiness, and by chance I found it. However, when I began to diffuse this practical method of life, I immediately encountered the second great problem of my life: THE WILL.

Marx discovered that all the evils of society originated with a bad distribution of food and drink; he wanted to teach the establishment of a correct system, by revolution. Scarcely 60 years after his death, this idea has become the guide of the greatest part of the world's population, yet one can see that social problems have not always diminished; on the contrary, they are continuing to grow, they are taking on a horrible aspect, they have escalated to the greatest degree, and all humanity trembles in uncertainty and lives in the fear of future war.

Health, liberty, peace, and individual happiness are always menaced. The hospitals and psychiatric clinics become establishments essential to city life, as temples and schools were in the past. The progress of medicine and medical paraphernalia are an indication of the increase in sickness and suffering; police reinforcement indicates the growth of criminality. This means that, although the theory of Marx has marvelously changed the structure of societies, it has forgotten the spirituality of man, the conception of the Universe, and its Will; that is, everything that is most essential.

If one practices macrobiotics, all incurable sicknesses are eliminated, and all uncertainties disappear with a single blow. The four physiological and biological scourges according to Buddhism: life, sickness, old age, and death, are problems resolved. Young students amuse themselves with their studies, adults succeed in their work, all become more and more happy each day, family life is gratifying, and all life becomes more and more interesting. If one lives correctly according to macrobiotics, all will go well and world peace will be rapidly realized. But the difficulty is that most people, especially the sick, don't have the will to hold to such a simple macrobiotic life. They lack will to such an extent that they prefer to submit to sickness and poverty, and are driven to crime. It is therefore necessary that the spiritual education, the education of the will, precedes the reconstruction of society. Even after this revolution is made, if one neglects the education of the will, one will add to the production of salaried conformists, slaves to their machines, a dependent race, which passes laws for playing with the machines for all who remain passive, robot observers and live blindly. Thus, in place of the creative spirit, it substitutes the spirit of imitation, because those who create themselves as well as their own destiny are very small in number.

The fundamental base of education is: (1) the self-control of health, and (2) the establishment of will. The first condition is resolved by applying the macrobiotic method. But, by what educative method can one fortify the will? This second condition is the great problem. What is the great secret?

What is Will (Levels of Will)

"To want is to be able," says a French proverb.

"Clear thought leads to saintliness," says a Chinese proverb.

In all times, all great men—the free men, the sages—have proclaimed the importance of the will. No one denies it; everyone agrees that this is so. Nevertheless, most of humanity fails to use the will in everyday life, and life ends tragically for man after having known only "the glory of the bindweed" (a short, ephemeral existence).

What are the reasons for this? What is the will? Are there many kinds or levels of the will? Are there other conditions than the will alone for changing the destiny of man?

Science keeps an absolute silence on these questions. This is normal. In the conception of Western studies, or rather techniques, the end of research is relative, limited, ephemeral, and physical. In other words, the focus is on the material world.

I pose these questions to the Far East, which has researched principally the infinite world—absolute, eternal, and constant; that is, the spiritual world. The response is the following:

1. The will is the progressive form of judgment.

2. There are seven levels of judgment and, therefore, seven levels of the will:

1. Mechanical, blind
2. Sensorial
3. Sentimental
4. Intellectual
5. Social
6. Ideological
7. Supreme

3. The seven levels reflect the natural development of life. For example, in a plant the development is from seed to sprout to stalk to branches to leaves to flowers to fruits. Judgment or will is vitality itself. However, the first six steps have value only in the relative, limited world. Only the seventh is valid in the absolute world, as well as the relative world.

4. Vitality, or the principle of development in nature, and the principle of the universe are the same.

5. Vitality increases by the mutual sympathy of the two elements, yin and yang: obscurity/light, humidity/dryness, dilation/compression, centrifugal force/centripetal force, etc.

6. The greatest mission of education is to make known the will (infinite expansion). When it is strong, it creates the man who has absolute health, who can "try without trying," "convince without speaking," "order the mountain to enter the sea," "conquer without fighting," "govern the strong with gentleness," "transmute the impossible into the possible," and "accept difficulties with joy."

Method of Education of the Will

Because the will develops naturally and freely through seven levels, an artificial and exterior education is useless. Even though animals do not go to school, they develop in a perfect and sane way. They lead a free life, without sickness, without worries, without poverty, without beautiful dresses, without scandalous pleasures. Instead of continuing the present system of education, it would be wise to discover a method of helping everyone to raise their judgment and change their thinking to one of deep appreciation and gratitude for their bosses, friends, enemies, etc. With this attitude, it doesn't matter what we do—we are happy any time anywhere, without the crimes and wars that men are practicing now. A small seed that has neither force nor arms, accepts conditions of darkness, pressure, cold, and dampness. Instead of complaining or blaming others, it uses these conditions as sources of energy. It is trampled on and eaten by insects and worms, but with each difficulty it fortifies itself and develops more and more. Thus, man can lead a free life and be at peace with himself if he accepts it as a grain does; but, on the other hand, if he looks for artificial ease, comfort, pleasure, assistance, wealth, and security, or if he has an Epicurian conception of life—in the current degraded sense of the word—he will weaken his natural vitality.

It is, therefore, important for education to give the opportunity and the chance to know the natural origin of health—to teach the way to achieve health in every sense of the word. This way consists of using the correct foods, combining them properly, cooking properly, and eating properly. As a consequence, one can discover and master by himself all the fundamental knowledge necessary to the social life of man, because judgment follows the process of its natural development. Those who, unhappily, have not received this education are the victims of natural selection, and will know only the suffering and difficulty of the world, and darkness of the seed and sprout. In time, many will fall in discouragement and become more and more unhappy, and manifest this unhappiness as criminals, slaves, and patients. The unhappy, the slaves, are the heavy burden of civilized society, and they can become the cause of war. The responsibility for the existence of unhappiness belongs to the low judgment of parents and educators. However, these difficulties and sufferings are the indispensable touchstone for those who have Supreme Judgment since only these social evils can transmute disparagement into will.

Education—Past and Future

During the 54 years that I have devoted to macrobiotics, I have spent more than 20 of them observing the educational programs of diverse Western countries. It is evident that their education is founded on scientific knowledge that has built their civilization. For the most part, the teachings are techniques intended to aid adaptation to life. This means that it is a materialistic education, adapted to the physical world.

From its origin, science has been a study of the physical world, following the research of Epicurus and Democrites. One finds systems of education founded on philosophy, religion, morals, and ideas, but these seem to be only accessories to the royal world of physics. Before the Renaissance, education was more blindly believing, mystical, and superstitious, but this approach was considered nonrealistic by the rational educational leaders that followed and was rejected. Consequently, this form of education is not concerned with metaphysics, and does not study spirituality, life, liberty, happiness, justice, memory, judgment, health, beauty, or art. It treats them only technically. Thus, modern education remains impotent before the increase in vandalism and cancer, which is the cause of 30 percent of deaths among the scholar-students of Tokyo and the appearance of 12-year-old diabetics! Likewise, it can only impotently remain with crossed arms before wars and massacres, and likewise before the situation in America where one person in ten is struck with mental disease at least once in his life. Neither Bertrand Russell, Schweitzer, Toynbee, the Pope, Sartre, nor any politicians can find a method that stops this miserable inhuman aggression, without parallel in history.

The leading articles in newspapers of the "civilized" countries speak morning and night of crimes, tragedies, and accidents. But they only expose the visible part of the great iceberg of crimes, and the incapacity of modern education. The proof is that all this is never, or hardly ever, found in the countries that have not made a great profusion of this so-called education. The more civilization and education develop, the more there are patients, unhappiness, and atrocious professional crimes. Modern armaments, the biggest inventions of science, have made possible great massacres and destruction on a scale never before realized in the history of humanity. The massacres of Auschwitz and the atomic bombs of Hiroshima and Nagasaki have been only preludes. These bombs, costing $1 million each, created by the scientist Oppenheimer, have killed 314 thousand persons on the battlefields of these two towns, and over the last 20 years they have slowly continued killing the survivors of the bombs.

Nevertheless, Vietnam is under bombardment, which costs more than $1 million a day! This condition of reality in Vietnam has moved and aroused the concerned Japanese youth to form the committee for "Peace in Vietnam," which is maintained and sustained by tens of thousands of students, Buddhists, Christians, Shintoists, and even politicians. Their action has sufficiently influenced the New York Times to make the appeal, "Can bombs bring peace to Vietnam?" Meanwhile, at the present time, the H-bomb is capable of slaughtering 100 million persons in one explosion and can at one blow wipe from the earth whole countries like England, France, and Japan! 100 thousand of these H-bombs are ready, of which the total capacity for destruction represents a slaughter of humanity 75 times over and the disappearance of all human civilization!

Contemporary world history began with "the India Company," the hunt for slaves in Africa, the landing in Goa and Hong Kong, and their occupation. The division and colonization of the countries of all the races by the whites made paradise completely disappear from the earth, which had been discovered by Kipling, Stevenson, and sailors who mutinied on the "Bounty." That is, the Westerners and the "civilized" have perpetrated scenes of slaughter and destruction throughout the world and are leading all humanity to its end, even though they believe they are capable of establishing a more beautiful and happier world. It is the clearest, actual result of scientific civilization and the education that it founded.

It is necessary to say that there are a few rare persons among the Westerners who have the capacity to self-criticize, and who have foreseen the end of humanity: Schupengrae, E. Carpenter, A. Carrel, etc.—bewailed and prophesied the tragedy coming and the end of Western civilization, of its education, in works such as, *The Failure of Western Science, Civilization: Its Cause and Cure,* and *Man, The Unknown.*

Lately, W. Heitler, current director of the Institute of Theoretical Physics of Zurich—like Einstein, he fled Nazi Germany and took refuge in free territory—has written and published a book under the title, *Man and Science*. Courageously, this wise man of modern physics insists on the necessity of forestalling humanity's demise, the biggest tragedy in history, produced by science and contemporary education.

One can make the following resume of his book: ...Scientific civilization, after extraordinary progress, has resulted in spiritual insanity. To save the world from this misery unparalleled on earth, and avert the ruin that approaches all humanity, one must before all save this science and this civilization from its stupidity and psychosis. Scientific civilization has been deluded from the start. Its research has only one end—occupation and dictatorship of the visible world, the physical world of matter, elementary particles, etc... It has forgotten that there was infinite spirituality and universal space beyond the world of limited and ephemeral particles. But what is most precious for humanity is this invisible world, the world of spirituality. Immediately, right now, we must stop all physical research and begin with all our force the dialectical research of the metaphysical world, the world of the spiritual civilization, the Order of the Infinite Universe! Here it is. The direction is given. The direction of the method that will save the contemporary generation, all humanity, all civilization, and all science.

Nevertheless, the research of metaphysics, spirituality, Will, Supreme Judgment, Happiness, Justice, Peace, and Liberty, and Infinite Life was the speciality of thinkers or sages of the Far East for 5,000 years. It is there the five great religions of man were born, but these religions have since become excessively antiquated mummies. Let us lay all this aside completely and start a new edition of the world, one that is neither physical nor metaphysical, but physical and metaphysical at the same time. It must provide the simplest and most practical method, which may be understood by all immediately, and is as applicable in the daily life of all races.

It is the new practical, physiological, and biological education.

Its unique instrument is practical dialectics: an amusing algebra, which resolves any difficult problem by employing yin and yang as the unknowns. Even children can understand it in an hour.

For 54 years, I have studied it; I have practiced it in my daily life; I have taught it; I have made many thousands of practitioners in all corners of the world. I have adequately confirmed this dialectic—otherwise called "the magic spectacles"—by my own practice. I have grown firm in my conviction by the confirmation that thousands of people of the scientific world, of the white race, have given me, after having practiced it like myself. I put the continuation of my discovery in the hands of the young people. Today, at the age of 74, I am calm and free, for the first time in my life. I receive each day letters of gratitude, soaked with tears, from unknown persons, from unknown countries, from all over the world.

The Education That Creates a New World: The World of Peace

Humanity has now ended the first chapter of its history, which, starting from the beginning of the Universe to the end of scientific civilization, comprises many thousands of years.

Its last page conforms to the prediction of the Apocalypse, in which all the predictions are realized, in order, from when the first angel sounds his trumpet to the seventh. Now is the beginning of the new world. The second chapter begins.

A new world begins with a new genesis.

The humanity of the first creation (that of Genesis) tried to adapt itself to the conditions offered by nature and to create a free and peaceful life, as the animals do: fish, insects, birds... However, man is born with a "thinking" brain, which makes the difference between other living beings. Why does only man have this brain that thinks? It is an important and interesting question, but I will not answer it here.

Because of this gift of thought, the manner of man's reply to nature's offerings follows two antagonistic processes of adaptation and development. One is harmonious adaptations; the other is the conquest of nature.

The first begins with innocent surprise and, passing through the mysterious, ends with the discovery of the Order of the Universe. It leads finally to the world of peace, infinite gratitude (ON), and universal identification.

The last begins with fear rather than surprise and takes the path of destruction, killing, and conquest by violence, all by way of hate.

This parallel between the faith of the Far East (the first process) and that of the West (the second) is very interesting because both, due to low judgment that dominates everywhere, have equally and normally produced lies, illusions, fantasies, wildness, hate, and malice. An example is the division between East and West that forms an extraordinary antagonism! Finally, the time has come for the East and West to come together. The West, whose end is conquest, came to conquer by violence the Far East, which considers adaptability as the superior way. These aggressive conquerors have run into a mutual collision of interests concerning each one's own profit, at the expense of the beautiful prey that is the Far East. Thus, at present the final scene of the miserable end of humanity is manifesting itself according to the prophecy of the Apocalypse!

But it is the time of the new beginning when all must be remade. The history of humanity is now at the first line of the first page of the second volume.

Let us re-establish a new world with our own hands: At first, re-education must be the way. This education establishes health first of all by its physiological and biological method. This is the setting in which the "will" appears: "a healthy spirit in a healthy body."

The education that will produce the new world, a free and peaceful world, begins at first with the creation of the healthy man. It is purely physical education, the reappearance and reproduction, physically and biologically, of a total process of 3 billion years of evolution. The product of the egg and sperm, after fecundation increases itself 3 billion times in 280 days. Then the baby grows only 20 times as much in the next 20 years. Therefore, these 3 billion years constitute a condensed process of primordial importance in the creation of man. I believe that it would be very suitable to count this period of 3 billion years as the biological unit of human evolution, as a generation of Life, or in other words, a "biological year."

"You are what you eat," said Francois Brillat-Savarin. During my study examining Far Eastern medicine, and during my 54 years of activity to diffuse it, I am more and more deeply and entirely convinced of the truth of these words, and I have arrived at this conclusion: if the nourishment is just, then the man is just.

Nevertheless, I had no way of knowing what was the correct nourishment across the unfolding march of evolution during 3 billion years on Earth. However, among the men who have practiced and been cured by macrobiotics with me, by which they had re-established their health, miracles produced themselves, one after another. They have had marvelous children. Even women who had never been able to have children have given birth to boys or girls, according to their desire. Childbirth has been without difficulty and very rapid. The children are in perfect health, particularly easy to raise, never catching cold. Everyone reacts with surprise when seeing them. Thus, I have discovered without a teacher, the principle of embryology.

Here are some examples:

1. The pastor of the Protestant center that is situated on the Ogoue River about 2 kilometers from the Schweitzer Hospital in the African jungle, M. Mayer, and his wife, had three young daughters (5, 3, and 1 years old). All three were so ill that the parents were very disturbed. They should have consulted the doctor who lived near the seashore, many hundreds of kilometers distance from them. Their nourishment consisted of only fruit preserves coming from France. We stayed with them for three months and, in this space of time, the children, like the parents, recovered their health. It was a joy to see these three happy children run in the African jungle, in Japanese kimonos!

2. A short time ago, a Japanese traveler, who was staying at a hotel in a German village near Schwartzard, had heard that there was a Japanese child in the village. Out of curiosity he enquired about the

family and went to visit them.

"Aha! (There's the Japanese child!)"

"Who is the Japanese father of this child? Where is he?"

"His name is Ohsawa; he is in the United States at this moment. He travels around the world each year. This child is mine after a long sterility. I have been able to have it while practicing macrobiotics, according to the books of George Ohsawa. The Ohsawa child is then a child of rice. Look, he is completely Japanese, isn't he?"

The traveler was completely amazed. As the mother told him, this child didn't seem German but Far Eastern. There are more than 120 children of this type in Europe and in the United States, the Ohsawa children, who were born thanks to macrobiotics. The largest number of them have Oriental features; a few have completely Japanese traits! Here is the key that completely resolves the secret of heredity and physiognomy. The characteristic common to all children born by macrobiotics is first of all absolute health, and next, they are wiser and more intelligent than the others, brothers or sisters. That is why Lima and I are accepted everywhere as their grandfather and grandmother.

The Nourishment of Expectant Mothers: I know of nothing more important for a human life and for society than the nourishment of the mother during the human embryonic period. It is the time of the fundamental construction of man's life. It is the period where the 3-billion-year process of evolution is condensed! I see nothing that has a greater influence on human life than this nourishment during the embryonic period. This is all that needs to be said concerning the fundamental education of man in the embryonic period.

The physiological and biological education of childhood and youth is of the greatest importance after the embryonic period. If one gives macrobiotic nourishment from this age, one will make boys and girls who fulfill the seven conditions of health. Moreover, whoever fulfills these conditions realizes by himself and for himself, a happy life. He becomes an independent man, who studies by himself. And a woman like this will be able to establish a happy family. She will devote herself to the construction of a happy and healthy society and country. If he finds one such woman in 10,000 (which makes 10,000 for 100 million), their country will become the country of liberty and peace. If he finds ten of these States in the world, peace on Earth will be maintained forever, and one will have seen atrocities, mass murder, and barbarous wars disappear (which don't even exist among animals).

If it is Peace—that is, the world where mass assassinations will have disappeared—that all humanity desires, then there is not any other education or method more simple to realize it.

By conferences and writings, everywhere in the entire world, I published this educative physiological and biological method for 54 years. And I have obtained more than sufficient confirmation of the efficacity; the examples of it are innumerable. They have been published in old reviews and books. However, here are a few of them:

1. Mr. William Dufty, 50-year-old American, holder of the highest honors from England, France, and Switzerland, former officer of aviation, hospitalized for more than ten years after the second World War, who no longer knew what to do with his body, which was like a living corpse, weighed 80 kilograms (176 pounds). He began to practice macrobiotics by following the directions in my books two years ago. He looks 20 years younger, losing 37 kilos in six months. In gratitude, he has decided to devote his life to macrobiotics. He has written and published *You Are All Sanpaku*, which required one year of work, but it has earned him a good reputation. He has declared that he will translate all of my works, in order to present them to the West.

2. Miss Cuilitz of Brussels, after having found a new conception of life through macrobiotics, has offered me a villa and apartments which are worth 20 million yen ($80,000).

3. An American girl, Miss Pletersky, of New York, saved by macrobiotics from a miserable death, saved for two years the money necessary for a pilgrimage to Japan, but she offered this money to the Vietnamese macrobiotics: this is living example of the transmutation of the conception of life.

4. Mrs. Teal Ames, an American actress, has quit her work,

which earned her 200 thousand yen ($800) each month, to devote all her fortune, and herself, to the establishment of a macrobiotic food distribution center, Chico-San Incorporated, in America. She worked on the production of a whole grain macrobiotic bread in this center, exactly like Cinderella (so well that a prince appeared and took her away in his pumpkin coach!).

5. "The Assassination by Zen": The macrobiotic front which had covered all the United States like an inundation, must face the most violent counterattack (from an article dated November, 1965).

Mrs. Simon, 24 years old, a young American artist, innocent as an angel or a child, was one among hundreds of thousands of Americans who threw themselves too fanatically into macrobiotics. The beautiful letters that she wrote me for the first time, just before her death, teach us vividly of her character.

At the beginning of February 1965, she began macrobiotics with her husband, and in nine weeks they were miraculously saved from terrible incurable sicknesses, caused by bad eating and drugs they had been using for ten years; for Mrs. Simon: neurosis, allergy, heart disease; for her husband: depression, tuberculosis, hardening of the arteries, narcosis. While following it, they added diverse diets to macrobiotics. So she died in October! It is well-known that often this type of woman-child, innocent and pure as a white pearl, lacks self-reflection and ends her life tragically. Her father was president of the lawyers association. He was against the "macrobiotics of the Rising Sun" and triggered off a massive campaign in the press, the magazines, and on the radio. The sale of my books was forbidden, the macrobiotic movement condemned, and Mr. Dufty of *You Are All Sanpaku* accused therefore as its editor, as well as Mrs. Irma Paule, the secretary-general of the Ohsawa Institute. This was an undoubted advance for the movement in America. This is not due to the radio, newspapers, and magazines where it was scandalized. But, on the contrary, because of this event, the number of macrobiotics in America has increased.

Mrs. Simon was an innocent and faithful woman and well-loved. But with her simplicity and honesty, she lacked judgment and deep thought like all Americans. Fatally, she came to this tragic end because she had no comprehension of the theory, although she was so enthusiastic about the practice.

Her case shows that "Philosophy without technique is useless; technique without philosophy is dangerous."

When one introduces a new idea or theory, the danger of accidents of this kind is inevitable. Theory without practice, philosophy without technique are useless. Technique and science without theory or philosophy are dangerous. It is the same with medicine, education, politics, industry, and agriculture if there is no principle— which means the First Principle: the Great Justice, the Principle of Life (health, beauty, happiness, liberty, justice); in other words, the "Order of the Infinite Universe." It is unbelievable but true that modern medicine ignores life! Politics has no other end than the monopoly of rights, profit-making, and the use of violence. Industry, commerce, and agriculture are deluded in considering profit as primary. It is especially unpardonable that agriculture, whose purpose is the production of the sustenance of life, has profit as an end and the unceasing increase in financial returns. The first constitution of Japan states formally that agriculture is the base of politics, and one of the three sacred rules in the formation of Japan established the National Order of Agriculture according to macrobiotic living.

The Unique State Called Happiness

Translated by Lou Oles from
the French review *Yin/ Yang*

The Tao is the Unique Way

What pleasure you seem to derive from drowning yourselves in the pool of sensory judgment! But do not fret—you are not alone. Even the president of the United States, the leaders of Soviet Russia, Bertrand Russell, and Gandhi have made extraordinary strides in the same realm.

Be grateful that until now you have not been made the victims of blind judgment like the seven million human sacrifices of the last war.

Up to the age of 27 years, I have not ceased to follow the narrow path; I am in a state of soul that is extremely calm and joyous: seventh heaven, the universe of infinite development cannot elude us... It is no longer out of reach.

Courageous men and women be strong! Step-by-step you can travel the unique way to the very summit.

The seven levels of judgment:

  7. Supreme, infinite
  6. Ideological
  5. Social
  4. Intellectual
  3. Sentimental

2. Sensory
1. Blind, mechanical

I. There are many methods for achieving a happy life.

Most of them come from the Extreme Orient and are spiritual. They run the gamut from ascetic religious training to the physical gymnastics of Yoga... there are hygenic and medical methods such as occidental science, yet there are few that have happiness as their final goal.

A Swiss scholar named Hilty has called his approach *Happiness*. It is motivated, however, by spiritual, moral, Christian culture that is difficult to apply consistently for most people with rare exception.

Methods like Marxism that promise the establishment of happiness in our material lives through social revolution or violent action are offering false hope. Many people know this already... the others will understand sooner or later.

We still have not found the scientific means to achieve happiness. On the contrary, what is called the happy life absolutely cannot come into being by way of science. The end of scientific civilization and the destruction of all of humanity can be the end results of thermo-nuclear war.

Nonetheless, you know that I do not make light of either social or scientific revolution. Many of you can vouch for the fact that I am likely to be in the forefront of either one. I openly declare that I am a man who does not oppose social revolution, civilization, or development in science. I have great respect for even an invention like the atomic bomb. And, I admire grandiose thermo-nuclear warfare.

I for one applaud both creativity as well as destruction. I would never hesitate to support any effort, however misdirected, if its goal were infinite liberty and eternal happiness.

I would not hesitate to offer all my admiration to even the medical conformist who earns his living by consuming the very life-blood of the most pitiable people on earth—ignorant slaves. Conversely, I proffer my sympathy and pity to those conformists upon such science and medicine.

Yet, I am content not to have played the game of these politicians, doctors, and revolutionists. To tell the truth, I was born a tragic character destined to end in tragedy at the head of a catastrophically sensational revolutionary movement. I inherited this character from my mother who died very young.

She passed away after having totally and gallantly followed a way of life based on the new science. I firmly maintain this spirit of my mother even now at the age of 70.

I believe that all men live with the spirit of their mothers as their principal driving force. The influence of the father is much less important.

Twenty years ago I wrote a long poem as a eulogy to my mother; I live in the spirit of that poem even today. For 70 years, all my words and achievements have been merely the actualization of that maternal essence.

In short, this has been the behavior of one who hungers and thirsts for Justice.

I live from morning to night (at night in my dreams) without being separated from my mother for an instant. I have lived at each instant for the realization of my mother's aims; this will continue to the end of my life.

My mother had lived her poor life believing with all her heart that scientific civilization, medicine, and modern hygiene were in actuality Justice. All Japanese, for that matter, believe that occidental science teaches Justice and the essentials of life (the very things they have come to take for granted in the Philosophy of the Extreme Orient). In reality, occidental methods are only techniques.

II. In traditional China, happiness depends on five conditions:
    1. Longevity—a long life
    2. Detachment from money: to not be influenced by wealth
    3. Security
    4. Cultivation of one's character and virtue
    5. Thinking unceasingly of ways to achieve the greatest and most marvelous thing, e.g.:

a. re-establishment of the health of one's body
b. re-establishment of order in one's family
c. establishment of a peaceful government
d. guiding the whole world towards Justice

Occidental happiness is quite another thing. Webster's large dictionary as well as the Larousse and the Littre Encyclopedia discuss happiness at length and reach surprising conclusions:

A. Happiness can never be achieved in this world.
B. It is a matter of luck.
C. Perfect happiness does not exist on this earth, etc.

My conclusion about occidental definitions of happiness is:

1. Wealth
2. Wealth
3. Wealth
4. Wealth
5. Wealth!

In short, money. Gold, silver, fortune, the treasures that Christ scorned have become the most important, precious things in the world. Thus, it is natural that science has become the most important study, that industry is most powerfully active. It is also natural that they could lead humanity into total war. In other words, intellectual judgment has replaced Supreme Judgment at the head of the list in the Occident.

I do not imply that intellectual judgment (the fourth level) is evil. If the Occident, however, were to reach social, then ideological and lastly Supreme all-encompassing judgment, science itself might produce even more miracles.

The Extreme Orient, which teaches Supreme Judgment from the very outset (it considers the other six as being of little importance), has been totally colonized by occidental civilization as we can plainly see.

In Japan, however, sentimentality (the third level of judgment) is remarkably well-developed. In matters of love, the guiding principle is the law of Supreme Judgment: all or nothing. Even in popular songs it is evident:

Fear not, I am yours even if it means plumbing the lowest depths of Hell! Paul Claudel, former French consul in the Orient, has left an extraordinary collection of traditional popular songs of this type.

Love in the modern world is either at the first (blind) level of judgment like that of amphibious plankton, or at the second (sensory) level like that of cats or dogs: it is no more than superficial, spontaneous, sexual.

If one does not have the emotional strength to live through this blind and sensory love, he cannot come to that of the sentimental (third) or intellectual (fourth) level.

To love is to make one's mate happy. The happiness of which I speak is really infinite liberty, absolute justice, eternal joy. This implies loving all—humanity, animals, vegetables. It is the Universal love described by Erasmus...love at the highest (seventh) level.

If you have not tasted the joy of loving one person with all your heart, with all your might, you cannot imagine the infinite joy of the love of which Erasmus speaks—Universal love or sadness. To understand, one has to have experienced the unbearable sorrow of being betrayed by his loved one.

In the spring, one falls in love—the miraculous product of the Yin-Yang polarization of the Sixth Heaven (see the Logarithmic Spiral). This should blossom into unlimited, infinite, absolute love. Un-

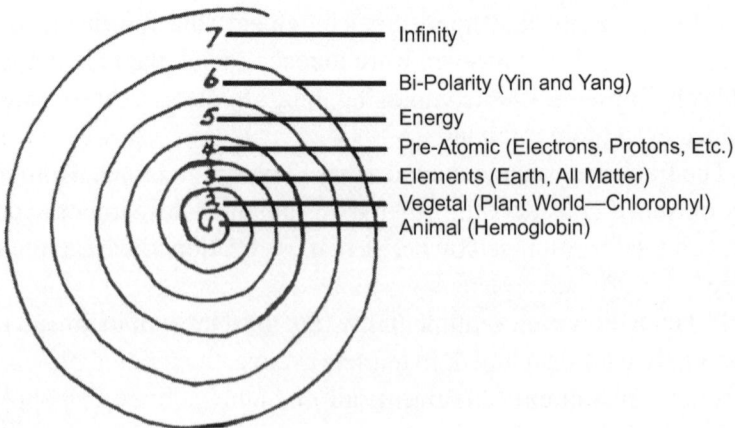

7 ———— Infinity
6 ———— Bi-Polarity (Yin and Yang)
5 ———— Energy
4 ———— Pre-Atomic (Electrons, Protons, Etc.)
3 ———— Elements (Earth, All Matter)
2 ———— Vegetal (Plant World—Chlorophyl)
1 ———— Animal (Hemoglobin)

fortunately, we arrest this development and concretize it at the blind or sensory level.

If you want to know the true character or judgment of a man, observe his behavior in love.

III. The condition that for me is the great, unique characteristic of happiness is not that of the Chinese definition, nor that of the Swiss, Hilty, of Descartes, Schopenhauer, or even Erasmus. Summed up it is to be a man.

It is the establishment of free will. To be a man signifies that one has mastered the logarithmic spiral of the Order of the Universe to which I have consecrated my whole life.

The different aspects of this world are due to the differentiation of the one aspect of the infinite or absolute. The origin of man is universal soul or spirit; the functions of which are memory, judgment, will.

The six levels that manifest themselves between the nondifferentiated world and the relative, differentiated world are the path or way of the eternal, logarithmic spiral in which man must accomplish a voyage in and out.

In other words, the true happiness of man is to explore precisely his native land—Seventh Heaven or Infinity. It is to clearly know the meaning of Oneness, to experience the fact that the soul is One, that all things in this world are indivisible despite the fact that human beings are apparently separate from one another and made up of billions and billions of cells. Here is the meaning of Unity, the concept of the identity of all humanity, the unification of the entire world. Having arrived at that point, one cannot distinguish others, and from then on, there is no separation. In the whole world, all are reunited in one, the term "others" no longer exists. There is neither strife, jealousy, rancor, nor envy. Therefore, if one experiences the sentiment of compassion or mercy toward others, he is an exclusive dualist!

Macrobiotic People Must be Inseparable

Those who breathe the same oxygen, who warm themselves at the same fire, who drink from the same source, who live and nourish themselves on the milk and blood of the same earth, who are born of the same womb are brothers and sisters. This brother and sister relationship, not a product of law or violence to begin with, cannot be broken by law or violence. Even more strongly so, the relationship between parents and children, between compatriots, between man and wife, between master and disciple, between intimate friends, cannot be broken during the length of one's life. Even if there is a clash of opinions or ideas, at the very most it is a contradiction peculiar to the first six levels of judgment. On the seventh level, there is no opposition and no need for separation.

In the realm of seventh judgment, there are neither possession, separation, despair, promises, duties, or rights. It is a world without contracts, the world of freedom, the world of the identity of self and others...the soul of millions of individuals. He who speaks in terms of opposition and separation is an opportunist and a dualist. He attests to his ignorance of the absolute and of infinity.

IV. Macrobiotic friends throughout the world. Friends who walk together on the road to infinite liberty, eternal happiness, and absolute justice, who are joined by a stroke of fortune that is extremely rare in this world, do not separate, do not abandon one another. There is no reason to discard a friend even if his comprehension is of the lowest sort because infinite liberty, absolute justice, and eternal happiness are one. There lies the realm of monism. If you abandon your friends, family, or teacher, it indicates that you are venturing into the world of opposition, the world of low judgment and dualism. Never separate, even if you are in conflict and struggling terribly with one another.

A brother is always a brother even after death. If one finds shortcomings in his friends, he can help them to change by seeking the cause of the problem. If you cannot make them see the light, your judgment has not yet reached the seventh level. You must redouble your efforts to improve yourself.

Gratitude is always gratitude—even for a glass of water or a bowl of rice. A debt of gratitude must be repaid ten thousand times over, or it will weigh you down forever. You are ungrateful, arrogant, exclusive. Master Ishizuka rescued me from a mortal illness. Consequently, I dedicated my life to saving ten million existences as a testimony of my gratitude: ONE GRAIN, TEN THOUSAND GRAINS. For me, ten thousand people represent the world. One grain, ten thousand grains is not, in reality, the mere discharge of a debt of gratitude. It is the realization of one's self in happiness, liberty, and justice. Only those individuals who follow the way of One Grain, Ten Thousand Grains, can become citizens of the land of infinite Liberty, eternal Happiness, absolute Justice.

V. These reflections on the unique state of Happiness are lengthier than I had wished. I am so clumsy in expressing myself. Furthermore, it is sad that the unique state of happiness should of necessity have to be described in a negative passive way, with phrases that begin with "it is not necessary," etc.!

The path of Macrobiotics and the Unique Principle to which I have consecrated my life is not a discipline that requires admonishments like "Thou shalt not" in the manner of Moses' Ten Commandments.

My path is without condition or limit. I have made a point of not using imperatives. The only condition or obligation or discipline that is more or less mandatory in macrobiotic practice is, CHEW THOROUGHLY.

Nevertheless, just as in a moral discipline, I tell you, "Do not abandon one another; there is no need to give up."

Obviously, this is a recommendation that is absolutely unnecessary for people with Supreme Judgment.

VI. This condition is actually useless in any case; there is no choice but to allow those people to leave who must.

The ones who abandon our monistic, unique path are dualists, inhabitants of the plankton and animal worlds. Slowly, one after the other, they struggle upward toward Seventh Heaven after having wasted several hundred million years. It is absolutely useless to advise them to imitate those with higher judgment. It is absurd and unhelpful. Such advice can be useful only to those who are near Seventh Heaven, who single it out like a beacon in the dark night.

Only Macrobiotics is Effective

To suffer from doubts as to the efficacity of Macrobiotics is the normal punishment for those who have not practised it seriously for ten years. One deviation erases the effectiveness of the preceding practice.

A man of low judgment often concludes that the Macrobiotic dialectic of the Unique Principle (the crystallization of Seventh Judgment) is a childish, simplistic concept. To him, it is suspect since it is not open to precise experimental study. This kind of opinion is precisely a reflection of simplistic, infantile arrogance.

Nuclear physics, at the conclusion of precise experimental study, has reached the conclusion that the fundamental unity of the Universe was formed out of protons, neutrons, electrons, etc. This is nothing but dualism or pluralism. And here we stand at the brink of mass suicide!

Here lies buried the tale of a long voyage on the road called Low Judgment.

Science suspects this. We can only hope that it will soon find its way to monism.

Note: This article was written by Mr. Ohsawa in 1963 and originally appeared in *The Macrobiotic Monthly, Vol. VI, No. 3* in 1966. It is as timely today as when it was first written and first published.

Conclusion

As you see, macrobiotic cures are very simple, but sicknesses are very complicated. None of them can be cured with one treatment or operation. They have many symptoms, may change form or location, and even evolve into other sicknesses. Some people say that bacteria and viruses are the only cause of disease. This belief is based in ignorance and superstition. Even total destruction of dysentery, tuberculosis, or syphilis bacteria, say, does nothing to change the patient's vulnerability to these or other diseases. It is impossible to live joyfully and happily at the expense of destroying some other so-called harmful form of life.

Other people emphasize heredity. This is either an excuse, an unwitting confession of incapable doctors, or a cover-up for ignorance. Furthermore, the act of destruction is cruel and violent. It reveals dualistic thinking.

Destroying living beings as a means to a peaceful life is a logical absurdity. If you see all life as one, whole and integral, then you understand destruction is a self-centered (schizophrenic) exploitation.

Creation is not a self-defeating, perverted process that leads man or other animals to mass slaughter.

A lion devouring a hare is first of all a rare occasion and one that teaches the hare to understand instinctually the way of this world. Note that the hare was becoming extinct for quite some time just because he did not know how to defend himself.

And the "lower" animals never wage all-out wars on each other.

Enough preaching about the superiority of man. The essential thing is the simplicity of following this oldest way of eating to heal any sickness without resorting to brutal destruction. This way of eating means understanding the biological and physiological basis of a happy and healthy existence. Study this basic concept seriously and carefully.

In both theory and practice, training in macrobiotic medicine with the aid of this book appears very simple. Actually, this oldest and most dynamic philosophy is quite inaccessible to the professionally educated Western mind. Absolute cure, I believe, comes not with the disappearance of symptoms but with the understanding of vedantic life and the unifying principle. By following satvic eating (*Bhagavad-Gita XVIII*), your life becomes an example of Krishna's teaching.

The way of eating is like raja yoga when it leads us to heal others. The only way to become man—healthy, happy, and free—is by helping others heal themselves, follow the way of eating, and become healthy, happy free men. Only then is your life a revelation of infinite freedom, eternal happiness, and absolute integrity. You will feel infinite love of all men, and you will be happy anywhere any time.

If you are a truly free man, all others should admire you, love you, and follow your ways, including your eating. Of the seven conditions of health, the first three refer to your physical state and the last four to your psychological state.

With the compass of yin and yang, you will find the just solution in harmony with the situation. No need for me to elaborate (necessity is the mother of invention). Without this compass, we rob and kill ourselves and each other.

You have discovered the compass, the *Weltanschauung* (universal wisdom). Assimilate it and master it so you can use it to cure any sickness and unhappiness. Your cup will flow over!

Giving

To eat is to live. To live is to give.

Remember the Order of the Universe: we of the animal world were born of the vegetal. Animals are converted vegetables, hemoglobin being a transmutation of chlorophyll.

Just as plants take their sustenance from the world of elements above them, so we in the animal world below feed upon and are nourished by the multitude of plant life.

What do we give?

All things exist for the purpose of giving life to higher beings. Just as the elements give freely to bring forth the vegetal, plants proliferate and give themselves to form the animal, so we of the animal world must follow their sublime example, in utmost harmony with the order of the Universe.

We must give.

Give freely. Give everything. Give all, with pleasure in the giving. To give that of which you are possessed of plenty is not a true gift. To give truly means to deprive oneself of something dear and necessary.

Accept

Accept everything. Illness is a blessing. A guarantee of order. Without order, there could be no disorder. Accept your illness with gratitude.

Accept misfortune as you do bonanza, knowing that it befell you because of some need or lack in you. Be grateful if your error or omission is pointed out, brought home to you. Accept war as you do peace, poverty like prosperity, foe like friend. He who embraces an enemy is the freest of all men.

You Must Change Your Life
> — Rilke, "Archaic Torso of Apollo"

You must change your life.

Such was the import of an archaic fragment of the Greek ideal upon a modern poet. Apollonian perfection once, but headless now, and without arms or legs.

"It is best not to be born," the sages sang, on the crest of a Golden

Age. And little wonder. Athenian intellect grafted reason and logic upon the natural tree of man, and a material philosophy flowered; the Western world is its fruit. The towers of Illium crumbled; Greek civilization declined; the glory that was Rome could not temper the barbarians' sword. The elixir of life is not found in rationality.

Heraclitus spoke out but who heeded him in a classic era when he said: The way up and the way down is one and the same, and wisdom is learning that all things are one.

God is day and night, winter and summer, war and peace, surfeit and hunger; and he takes various shapes, just as fire, when it is mingled with spices, is named according to the savor of each.

What is at variance agrees with itself. It is the opposite that is good for us.

Cold things become warm, and what is warm cools. What is wet dries, and the parched is moistened. It scatters and it gathers. It advances and retires.

Good and evil are one.

The 20th Century is materialism's legitimate heir-at-law. The Hellenic tradition in the West obtains today, despite the continuing lessons of two millennia: strife, warfare, bloodshed.

Reason and logic are yet enthroned, but, in truth, over whom do they rule? What is their domain and where are their subjects? Where can one single subject be found? Better the old pantheon of capricious gods meddling in the affairs of men than materialism's gross, life-denying aims. Industrialization, science, technocracy, and progress are some of the new gods' names, and each bears its own built-in mechanical Vulcan for forging mankind's glittering new chains.

Freedom

Detach yourself from anything and everything not actually necessary for your bare existence. *Vivere parvo*. Do not depend upon anything or anybody. Depend upon yourself alone.

So long as you carry a tin of aspirin in your pocket you are not free. Aspirin is no cure, only a palliative. Each five grains of aspirin you take destroys a million brain cells. Take no drugs of any kind.

A headache is the first signal of a yin imbalance in your body's chemistry. Aspirin, another yin, increases the disorder. Yangize yourself, instead. Stop drinking for a day. The headache will disappear, and your system welcomes the return of its natural balance.

Be Macrobiotic!

All doors are closed to you. There is no place to hide. The solution is simple: become macrobiotic.

"If the doors of perception were cleansed, everything would appear infinite."—William Blake. Be macrobiotic. The essences of all things shine and sing; edges are sharp and defined, yet all is one. The quantity and quality of life enhanced—*vistavision*—a unique awareness. The senses receive truly. How pure and perfect is the smallest thing and its counterpart, the Yin and the Yang, magnificent! The liberty of imagination and impulse, the depth and breadth of reality, the infinite, once glimpsed, never forgotten.

Half-beings become whole. Forever one foot in the infinite.

See with the brightening glance, know the dancer from the dance. Impressions are clear, clean, precise, and joyous, the senses receive and transmit freely; the memory is liberated. The ruts of old thought patterns are erased, and direct action follows without jolt or interference. Whatever you desire is yours. But, note that your desires have changed.

All is clear. Clarification of reality: man's freedom. Absolute truth, absolute justice reigns, and no falsity exists. You will judge for yourself everything forever after. No law, causal or man-made, will command your adherence until you test it in the light of your changed self. Old truths are re-examined and discarded if false; the new truth is infinite.

When the doors of perception are cleansed: reality, sharp and clear...and perfect. Color is infinite; all things radiate it, and man's history lies plain upon his face. There are no secrets; light and dark are interchangeable, are one; the cosmos is in flux, expanding and receding tides of air.

Be macrobiotic!

The Secret of Macrobiotic Medicine

Mr. Chitarangia is 63 years old. He is one of the revolutionaries of India. He was jailed several times. He has a strong will. He practised a pure vegetarian diet (nothing but vegetables, fruits, and water) for 23 years in order to improve his health and mentality.

After studying macrobiotics with me, 2 hours every day for 10 months, he changed the diet to the macrobiotic diet. He is observing the strict macrobiotic diet now, which consists of 10 ounces of millet, less than 5 ounces of vegetables, salt, and sesame oil. He doesn't urinate more than twice a day. It is I who worry about his too-strict observation of the diet. One night, Lima did palm diagnosis on his shoulder while I was talking with him.

He said, with uneasy attitude, "Why do you put your palm on my shoulder? If it is for the healing, please stop it."

Lima answered, "No, I am checking where the sickness is and how your sickness is improving."

After that he was contented. He didn't want any symptomatic cure because he knows his sickness is the punishment of the Order of the Universe. His attitude is the secret of macrobiotic medicine.

There is no real cure except self-reflection, that sickness is my fault. Punishment for the fault must be accepted even though such punishment may seem unjust. No excuses. Even when you are resented, envied, or scolded by mistake or misunderstanding, you should not make any excuses because there is no excuse in nature. (Only man makes excuses.) There is no need to excuse the Order of the Universe because it is perfect and makes no mistakes. Justice reveals itself.

One who excuses does not understand the Order of the Universe at all. Man was born in the world of Freedom, Love, and Peace, where the Order of the Universe is called Justice. We are living without awareness of the Order. This order can neither be disturbed nor distorted. Millions of tons of bombs may destroy all the towns on earth, and make the sky dirty for awhile. However, nature will clean up the sky again.

Man creates dirt, poisons, and unhappiness. Man exhales poisonous gas every 16 minutes. He secretes 2-3 pounds of stinky liquid and waste every day. Some of them are brave enough to cause war, sickness, and social violence. Most of them consume 30 million pounds of matter during their lifetime. The destruction of man is huge and enormous. However, it is allowed.

God made man to be destructive and create unhappiness. However, God also made man to be aware and observe infinite Freedom, eternal Happiness, and absolute Justice. Man's destruction is limited and infinitesimally small compared with the greatness of the Wholeness—God. Man's work is to join God's creation. Other things such as to make money, business, fighting, sickness, etc. are only things to lead man to unhappiness. Once you understand the exactness and justness of the infinite universe and smallness of man, you will not dare to excuse any of your own faults.

Mr. Doger, the younger brother of Mr. Chitarangia, was jailed on September 10th because he marched at the head of the protesting demonstration against killing cows. He has been in jail since then for over 100 days without any court action. By his status and money, it is easy for him to be released. However, he is a man of no excuse. He is staying in an uncomfortable jail without any complaints or excuses while giving me permission to stay in his marbled mansion and to use his luxurious car. Furthermore, he is helping me to get status so that I can stay in India permanently.

Many famous people come to see him everyday in jail to salute him. However, he doesn't ask anybody to get him out of jail. He is the man of "no excuse."

These two brothers know the Order of the Universe, which has absolute justice. They have complete faith in the Order. This faith and this attitude of "no excuse" is the secret of Macrobiotic Medicine.

Part 4

Experience with Macrobiotic Medicine

My Graduation Certificate of Macrobiotic Medicine

I Tumbled Seven or Eight Times in Twenty Hours

We left our home to visit Lima's parents on September 7th at 3:30 p.m. Her father was 80 and her mother was 79 at that time. This was the first occasion I had to visit her parents. We knew that they would miss us when we left Japan if we did not visit them first. However, it was not only for that purpose that we went. I had a desire to quietly write some articles before I left Japan and could do so at their home.

It was already dark when we arrived at Kusakabe station. We bought presents for her parents and food for our three-day stay. Then we continued the trip toward their home by taxi.

They welcomed us warmly. I went to bed early so that I could get up at two o'clock in the morning to write.

The next day (September 8th) at one o'clock in the afternoon, I noticed pain in my intestine. I thought to myself "this is it!" I took a teaspoonful of dentie, and another one. In all, I took five teaspoonsful of dentie, but the pain did not stop. "This should be the final attack," I thought. The pain continued 20 hours, starting again at seven o'clock in the evening until nine o'clock the next morning. During this time, I tumbled and fell down seven or eight times.

This type of pain had begun three months ago, around the middle of June. It had occurred once or twice a day regularly. Each time, I had taken a half-teaspoonful of dentie (0.5 grams), and it had stopped miraculously. I had been taking dentie because I thought the cause of the pain was yin. Why did I think the cause was yin? I had received a gift of two melons in the middle of June. Nobody in my home had dared to eat them, so I had greedily eaten both of them. They were delicious.

I had the same experience before this. Thirteen years before at summer camp, I had received many melons as a gift. One of the melons started to spoil. I couldn't let it spoil, so I ate it—a big one. Severe diarrhea began that night. I went to the bathroom 30 times in one day. I looked like a skeleton the next day. I was able to stop the severe pain by using ginger hip bath. I was scheduled to go to summer camp at Otu, but my body looked terrible. It was not a human shape. I had to recover my form in one day...but how? I took a strong yang and waited three to four hours until I was thirsty. When I felt thirsty, I bore the thirst for two to three more hours. Then I drank as much rice soup as I could. I continued to drink it even on the train going to Otu. When I arrived at camp, nobody realized that I had had severe diarrhea the day before.

Since that time, whenever I ate melon I had a stomach ache. This forced me to stop eating melons. This time I allowed myself to eat a melon because 13 years had passed since the last experience. That was my mistake. After I had two melons, I experienced a pain in the stomach, no appetite, and a sick feeling.

There was severe pain every day. Each time, I stopped it by taking dentie. Sometimes I would eat a hamburger at a high-class restaurant to keep the use of dentie from becoming a habit. This stopped the pain miraculously. Since then, I ate hamburger and egg whenever I felt pains and was away from home. However, I continued to use dentie in my home.

Sometimes the pains would start when I was lecturing. When this happened, I would press my lower abdomen—forcefully—with my right hand, and nobody noticed that I was in pain.

At any rate, I thought that the cause of this pain came from yin.

I Had Cancer!

I started to worry when I had pains every day, even when taking such a strong yang as dentie, hamburger, or egg. (Hamburger is typical of the German cuisine that built a yang Germany and made possible a million dollar income from the practice of acupuncture by some 300 practitioners.)

What is the matter? Why doesn't dentie or hamburger stop the pain? This may be fatal for me, I thought to myself.

I had a cancer, which I had kept secret. When I was 25 years old, I helped Or. Okabe's touring clinic. He diagnosed my stomach as cancerous because there was a big lump inside the stomach. At the age of 18, I was not only tubercular but had diseases of the heart, kidney, eyes, teeth, and intestines, in addition to hemorrhoids.

The curing of my cancer was the next aim when I had cured the tuberculosis. Since then, I had been fighting with cancer for 40 years without telling anyone. However, I was always afraid that I might die of cancer at any time, and people would laugh at me or macrobiotics.

My physique as a boy was so yin that I looked like a girl. I was writing very sentimental poems at that time under the pen name of "Ruisei" (meaning Tearful Voice!). Therefore, I tried hard to yangize myself by taking much salt for 40 years.

Now, I thought I had failed. It was the beginning of July. I was shocked when I faced the thought. There was another reason why I thought this way. Since January I had started to eat sweet things, including fruit and to drink beer in order to find a cure for gray hair for my best friend, Mr. Itoga. I was confident that Mr. Itoga had never eaten much meat or fish to cause his gray hair. Something must be the matter with my dietary teaching. I decided to find out what was wrong.

Then I started to take a little yin food. However, my greatest shortcoming is going to extremes, greediness. I am never satisfied until I reach the bottom. I will eat a boxful of sugary pastry in one day instead of one each day. Then I will eat fruit and drink beer. I could eat 10 sugary cakes, 12 bowls of red bean moti custard, or 24 moti cakes at one time. No one could exceed my greediness, and yet I never recognized this fault in myself.

I did the same thing this time. Whenever eating yin foods I was not moderate but extreme. Disregarding Lima's surprise and worry, I ate candy, fruit, and beer until I tired of them. I believed that greediness is a sign of God. I admired greediness. I thought greediness was a symbol of a great man.

I grew up in a poor family. My stomach was never full. Until the age of 20, I was always hungry. Therefore, nothing would happen when I ate a lot of candy, fruit, or beer because I did it only once in three to five years. (My advice: Always be hungry until you are 20 years old. This is the secret of success.)

Now I have broken my 40-year-old commandment for one year. I ate sugar and honey. I might have tapeworms. I thought so when the pain began again.

I Seek the Cause

As I said before, my severe pain began at one o'clock on the afternoon of September 8th. Lima's brother came to visit me, and I talked with him without showing any pain. Because he didn't realize the pain I was in, he stayed until after dinner. As soon as he left, I lay down on the bed. However, I couldn't even moan because Lima's parents were sleeping next to our room, separated by just a thin paper sliding door. I had to suffer the pain all night without making a sound. Lima's palm therapy did not work at all this time.

I tried to vomit at ten o'clock. Nothing came up. I tried again at eleven o'clock, and gall bladder juice came up. But no stomach juice came up, which is common in the case of cancer. "Then I do not have cancer. This may be a tapeworm."

Pain became severe at 12:30.

"What do you think the pain is, Lima? Do you know the cause?"

"No, I don't understand at all"—she is almost crying.

Two o'clock—more severe pain.

"Lima, how long will this pain continue? If this pain lasts for more than ten hours I will be finished. However, you can't help me anyway. Please go to bed. This is not a yin sickness because so much dentie doesn't work."

Lima soon went to sleep. I tried to sleep but couldn't because the pain was too severe to sleep. Dentie doesn't work; then this is not a yin sickness. This must be a tapeworm... a big worm... many worms. It must be like a snake because it gives me such a strong pain. Is this possible? I thought about the cause as I struggled with the pain.

What is the cause of this pain if it is from too much yang? Hamburger or egg? I ate one bowl of brown rice in the morning, two eggs at lunch the day before yesterday. Yesterday I ate brown rice and red beans in the morning, red bean rice and miso soup for dinner, and a few rice cakes for a snack.

Three o'clock. I twisted my body into all types of positions but could not relieve the pain—it did not diminish. My body was sweating, but I did not have the strength to get up and get a towel.

I kept thinking about this sickness, and I still didn't understand the cause. There is no such thought as "I don't know" in the Unique Principle, because yin and yang judgment is the lowest judgment and starts 24 hours after birth.

Most pains are up and down—strong and weak—but my pain had continued constantly for more than ten hours. I wondered. This is neither a stomach cramp nor cancer. Is this a tapeworm? I woke up Lima and asked her.

"What do you think is the cause of this pain?"

"I don't know. The sweets you ate were less than one-fifth of what a normal person eats, and only a half-bottle of beer. I don't think that is the cause."

"If this pain continues two to three days, I will die."

"We must stop this trip."

"Please find out the train schedule to Tokyo."

Time passed... five o'clock, six o'clock, seven o'clock, eight o'clock.

Macrobiotic Medicines are Yang

On September 9th, we hastily bid farewell to Lima's parents and went to the station. It was fine weather (yang); I carried a heavy suitcase (yang); and jumped on the departing train (yang). At that moment the pain disappeared.

At the next station I said to Lima, "How wonderful! I am cured."

"?"—Lima had nothing to say. She wondered.

"I said, I am cured."

"???"

"Finally, I found the cause. It is not by yin."

"Then hamburger or egg?"

"No, no... too much yang accumulated over 40 years."

"Why, too much yang!"

"Yes, too much yang. What a wonderful thing. All along I have been thinking that I was too yin and trying for 40 years to make myself yang. As a result, my constitution has completely changed. What a wonderful thing."

Lima was still puzzled. I recalled the efforts of 40 years and of the strange sickness in June. Now I had found the cause. I had no more worry about pain. However, I must make sure my judgment is right; I must try a vermifuge. If a tapeworm doesn't come out, I am sure that the cause of my sickness is yang. The next question that entered my mind was: What kind of treatment do people receive from modern medicine when they have such severe pain?

"It is clear to me. Now I'd like to go to a hospital and discover their treatment."

"Then Junten Hospital is the best. I went to that hospital for 15 years, though all my doctors may not still be there," said Lima.

I bought "Santonin" in Tokyo and drank it all, against Lima's advice. The quantity I drank was three times the recommended dosage. Then we went to a coffee shop where I ordered cake and tea. I had to eat it while Lima was in the bathroom because she was against my doing this.

Then we arrived at Junten Hospital, one of the most famous hospitals in Tokyo. There were many patients waiting all over the building—the waiting room, the reception room, and even in the lobby. How many people there were suffering from sickness each day! They were waiting to be cured. How many of them will be cured?

I sat down among them. Strangely enough, I had no pain. I wanted to eat something yin, but Lima was there. A receptionist called my name without much wait because Lima had admitted me as an emergency patient. A young doctor checked me thoroughly, especially my abdomen. I told him my symptoms.

"What is it? Is it cancer? The pains came to me either in hunger or after meals."

"I don't know yet."

"Is this a tapeworm?"

"I don't know. You had better be hospitalized. Anyway, I will give you an injection."

"What kind of injection?"

"Something good for you."

It is public custom to receive unknown injections. I followed in the same manner. It was yin anyway. I needed such yin.

I paid the 50-cent fee and, after stopping to see a movie, returned home. As soon as I got home, I lay down on the bed to rest, because I was tired after suffering for 20 hours from the severe pain. I knew that sleep was the best medicine. I would find a good remedy after I woke up. I woke up at three o'clock in the morning because the pain had begun again. Should I drink radish drink No. 1 or No. 2 or something else. However, there is no yin medicine in macrobiotic medicine because everyone has yin sickness. Yin foods are abundant in the markets: apples, cake, beer, sake, coffee, tea, potato, banana, whisky, champagne, rum, chocolate, etc. Now those poisons were medicine for me.

Chinese Medicine and Whiskey

The pain continued...four o'clock...five o'clock...though it was not as severe as the last time. There was, however, no yin food or drink available.

Dr. Kawachi came at eight o'clock. I asked him for a diagnosis of my pain. He was an expert of Chinese medicine but could not find the cause of my pain immediately.

"How do you treat such cases by Chinese medicine?"

"First of all Hanka-Shashin drink, then Taiken-Chu drink."

"What is that?"

He told me that both were made from several Chinese herbs and contain five grams of dry ginger each. They are extremely yin. What a wonderful diagnosis of Chinese medicine. I asked him to prescribe both. (Communist China is a great country because she authorizes Chinese with the Western medicine. Japan stopped the authorization of Chinese medicine and became one of the sickest countries of the world.)

"Shall I give you an injection?"

"That is a yin of Western medicine, isn't it? It is poison for the nervous system. Okay—we can find out which is more yin, Eastern medicine or Western medicine. I had an injection in the hospital yesterday, but it wasn't yin enough."

He gave me a shot of pantpon-atropine—extremely yin. There was no reaction after five minutes, eight minutes, ten minutes and fifteen minutes.

"I will give you another one."

Finally the pain was gone, 12 minutes after the second injection.

There were no side effects. I was feeling very well.

"What do you apply in macrobiotics for this condition?" he asked me immediately.

"Whisky," I replied right away.

"Okay, I will go buy some."

"Wait, It must be pure—the best whisky. Black and White Scotch."

Lima brought me the Hanka-Shashin drink. It had a good smell of ginger. I tasted a little. It was very good, delicious, wonderful. When Lima hurriedly stopped me, I had already drank a half-day's quantity. I drank the rest when Lima left for the kitchen.

Next Lima brought me the Taiken-Chu drink. This had the same smell of ginger. It was also delicious. I drank it all when Lima wasn't near. The quantity was enough for ten people. I was very comfortable.

Two to three hours later Dr. Kawachi brought me the whisky, I drank half of the bottle without stopping. I had never tasted so delicious a beverage, even though this was not the first time. What a wonderful thing to have a sickness that will allow me to drink such delicious medicine—whisky.

I would like to drink another cup of Taiken-Chu drink.

The Tapeworm Like a Dragon

My 100 days of stomach pain had been cured by Chinese herbs and whisky. It was a dream or a miracle. September 9th was a memorable day for me.

Sometime in October, Lima asked me: "Did anything happen to your stomach?"

"What?"

"Your stomach, of course."

"Nothing."

"It's like a dream."

"Yes, it is a dream."

"I was afraid because you said a big tapeworm, like a dragon, was causing the pain."

"Yes, it was a tapeworm—like a dragon."

"You tell a lie. When did it come out?"

"Didn't you see it when it came out. I saw it. It was a big one with a black head and blind. It was a dragon called human wisdom or ignorance."

"Ah! I understand now."

"It was a frightening experience."

"Yes. I was afraid."

"I, too, was scared."

"Then is whisky the wisdom of God?"

"Yes, that's right. Isn't it wonderful?"

"Then I will go out and buy some."

"That is a good idea."

"But even if it is good, it will be bad to drink too much."

"Yes, it is bad to drink too much; one bottle a month is okay."

"You had three bottles within three weeks—since September 10th. Is that not too much?"

"Not for me. It was medicine to me. Do you understand?"

"You are like a warrior who killed a big snake by giving it sake. Isn't that true?"

"That's right. The mythology is mine. The big snake is human ignorance!"

"You may have a purple dragon next time because everyone will give us whisky."

I recalled Mr. Tenko, a famous religious leader who liked sweet cakes. Everyone would give them to him, and he became sick from it.

A leader must not be particularly fond of any one thing. Otherwise, he will be killed by what he likes.

"The best thing is to like everything."

"Are you really cured?"

"Don't worry. I am cured."

"It is wonderful. It is hard to believe."

"Yes, this is the medicine of macrobiotics' Unique Principle and Natural Hygienics. How marvelous."

Pears, Grapes, and Beer

My story must go back. I left Tokyo and went to Eda with Lima, by train, on September 11th—four days after we had gone to visit Lima's parents. When we were leaving Tokyo, I ate about 13 ounces of grapes. In my bag, my secretary had put two bottles of whisky—though I had asked for only one.

"Good boy!"

"It is too much. One bottle is enough," Lima said. I pretended not to hear her, and I started to drink the whisky. By midnight, one bottle was empty. At the Eda station, nobody came to welcome us. I had to carry my heavy bag, but had no pains. I was feeling good. On the way back to Tokyo the next day, I ate several pears (which I had received as a gift), grapes, and drank some beer also.

My Life in Forty Years

I was saved. My 100 days of pain was like a dream. Why had I suffered so much? It was due to my black tapeworm (ignorance). I had tried to "yangize" for 40 years. Around the age of 30, salt would come out on my face in the summertime. I was taking too much salt at that time. No one could duplicate that. Several people tried but failed.

I started to reduce the salt intake around the age of 35. Before that, I was too salty a man. At the age of 27, I was manager of a trading company in Kobe. They handled one percent of all Japanese exports at that time. The main export items were silk, pearl buttons, and general merchandise. There were 30 employees. With the exception of two, all employees were younger than me. Therefore, I was considered a sharp and unusual youth by financial and business groups in Kobe. The manager of the First Bank of Kobe offered me an unconditional letter of credit. I was surprised that this amount of credit was given to me.

To make a long story short, I was an aggressive, vigorous businessman. I had no patience with delay. I kicked out a lunch tray when it was served five minutes late. I tore up a typed copy in front of the typist if it had a misspelled word. I kept three typists and 30 employees busy the whole day. Each year, I had to go abroad to resolve claims or recover unpaid accounts. During these times, my experiences paralleled Mr. Fukushima's dream (see *Macrobiotic Guidebook for Living*)—collision at sea with an English ship on a stormy night in the Bay of Biscay—or the time I was almost killed in a foreign port after taking too much drink.

When I was 35, I quit business and began to re-establish a macrobiotic association in Tokyo. I was more yang than ever. All of the members of the macrobiotic association were very much afraid of me. Miss Morivame, my secretary, would give me delicious yin cooking every day—or a sweet potato (it was my favorite food during my childhood). Even so, I was still extremely yang.

I separated with my wife because she didn't agree with my spending all our money on macrobiotic activity. Although she was an excellent secretary when I was in business—she wrote English and French, could type and take stenography, understood music and art, and thus was a good companion on a foreign business trip—she couldn't bear to be poor or hungry.

A yang man will go after women or drink if he has no wife. He will seek the company of several women if he has money. Although I earned much money from stock investments, all my money went to printing and advertising macrobiotics. In addition, I had no time at all to do anything else. I got up at two o'clock in the morning and studied French, Greek, and Latin; furthermore, writing articles on macrobiotics for magazines, corrections, and mailing were my job. No money, no time saved me from running after women and liquor at that time.

Why Was I Saved?

I was saved because I had led a disciplined life of yangization for 40 years. The cause of my sickness: My constitution had changed from yin to yang, completely, after 40 years of yangization with salt. Without knowing this, I took more yang food when the sympathetic nervous system (which is yin) resisted the yang. This was the cause of my symptomatic pain. When I ate sweets, beer, or fruit, they triggered this resistance or violence and finally exploded on my last trip to Lima's parents. The cause of my sickness was my ignorance of not knowing I was taking too much yang. I was extremely yang. Then it was natural that I was saved by extreme yin such as pantponatropine, morphine, ten times one person's amount of Chinese yin herb drink, and a half-bottle of whiskey.

Why was I saved?

1. I never gave symptomatic treatment until I knew the cause.

2. It was an excess yang sickness (excess yin leads to death).

3. This world is yang. Animals are yang. Man is the most yang

animal. (Man's civilization and war is its proof!) Therefore, too much yin is death.

4. Man never dies from too much yang food, because the relative world is formed by a binding power (yang). However, because animal foods (yang) contain much sulphur and phosphorus (both are yin), animal yang will change into yin and will bring partition and destruction.

5. Yang from vegetables, fire, salt, and activity will not harm us because at the extreme yang, we will have good judgment (yin). [Editor's note: This statement will not apply to persons who have been heavy meat-eaters or drug-users. Their judgment is too rigid to realize when their sickness is caused by too much yang, especially salt. Therefore, for most Americans, it is better to modify Mr. Ohsawa's above conclusions—4 and 5. Instead, avoid extreme usage of salt.]

6. Within the yang factors mentioned in 5, activity is the safest. When you have big yin such as lack of time and money, yangization will not harm you. There are more reasons, and you must find them for yourself.

7. The last and most important reason is that I am naive and humble; in other words, I am yin. I accept everything. I don't try to escape from anything, even tragedy, trouble, or unhappiness, because I know that I have attracted such unhappiness or trouble. Yang attracts yin and vice-versa. I know well that I am a powerless, ignorant, ephemeral creature in this world. This naivety and humbleness finally saved me. I was saved miraculously. I didn't ask anyone how to cure myself—my judgment saved me. I am happy. What a wonderful thing that I—this ignorant man—was saved. I am a happy man.

There is Nothing in This Story

One girl, out of 50 who heard my story, didn't understand the importance of the story. She said, "I can't understand why George Ohsawa didn't realize that he was too yang. Even I knew that."

I was shocked by hearing this. I have learned many things from this experience, as I mentioned under the last heading. The most important lesson to be learned is that ignorance, rigidity, and low judgment is the cause of all unhappiness or sickness. Such ignorance, rigidity, and low judgment will change to the highest judgment by the macrobiotic diet. It took me 40 years of strict discipline to learn this.

I am very grateful that I stopped eating sweets 40 years ago. The reason people don't stop eating things that are bad for them, even when they know better, is because of low judgment. I found the way to improve judgment. What a wonderful experience.

<u>Some readers, who have low judgment, will imitate this experience and eat grapes, pears, or beer; and they may die from it. Please don't forget that I used this therapy once in my life. This type of therapy is good only for persons, like myself, who have yangized over a period of 40 years.</u>

This is my graduation certificate of Natural Hygiene (Macrobiotic Medicine). I will prove that this certificate will save thousands of people in the world.

Postscript

Once upon a time, there lived a boy. His parents died when he was young. He was left alone in this world, but he remembered what his mother told him when she died.

"Go East, then you will come to an ocean. Cross the ocean, then you will come to a mountain. The top of the mountain will be clouded, but climb that mountain without hesitation or giving up. There is a happy land at the top of the mountain. I will see you there."

He did as he was told and began to climb the mountain. However, the top of the mountain was always far away. He fell down many times. He clung to the roots of trees and rocks. He kept on through rain, storm, snow, and wind because he wanted to see his mother. His clothes tore, and cold and hunger tortured him. Finally, he fell upon the snow and lost consciousness. When he awoke, he was with a beautiful goddess. There were many flowers, grass, and trees everywhere. There was a big castle at the end of the grass road.

"You have reached the top of the mountain," said the goddess. "This is Seventh Heaven, World of Absolute Justice, Eternal Freedom, and Infinite Happiness." Then she pointed toward the castle, where a lady came riding a white cloud.

"She is your mother," the goddess said.

"Oh, my mother!"

He Was Blind, Until He Opened His Third Eye

He was a simple, honest workman. He was an atheist; he didn't know God. He became very sick and unhappy. He was operated on 19 times in several years—in vain, quite in vain. In seeking a cure, he discovered vegetarianism, but this gave him no relief. Later, he had a chance to listen to me during my lectures in Paris. He observed my directions correctly, according to Oriental philosophy and the Unique Principle, and he was soon cured. He has lived macrobiotically for the last two years, becoming happier and happier. I don't remember him, because he was one among the thousands of people I met in Europe. He attended a few of my lectures and read my books in French. There are thousands of people like this in Europe and more in Japan. Being very simple, honest workmen without power, they do not protest against the murderers who drove them into hell—so cruel, so brutal, and so bloody. They stay silent. They are grateful only to God, and they disappear, continuing their slavery, their terrible fate. One among ten thousand will write me of his happiness. This is the case of Mr. I., the author of the following letter that I received at New Horizon Camp recently. This is his first letter.

I wrote him in reply to find out in how many weeks he was relieved from his suffering, and to ask what more he wants of me. I asked also that he leave his business and become a representative of the Divine Art for all those who are suffering as he had suffered. He should be the one who has, and who will receive, everything in abundance. He didn't know that he was in the midst of paradise or the Kingdom of Heaven because he was blind. Now his third eye is open, and he realized what the Kingdom of Heaven is and its Justice. He was, and is, and will be, always in the House of God, forever. No one can escape from the House of God. Hell or the House of Satan exists only in the imagination and in the body of a blind man. Then one cannot see Divine Law or Divine Justice.

I am very happy to receive such a letter. Even one like him, among millions, encourages me and confirms my own way.

– Fontenay aux Roses, 8/15/60

My Dear Master Ohsawa:

A spark just came out and here the light will shine! God sent me to tell you my personal little history, in relation to a deep sickness that lasted several years and of which I am cured today, thanks to the macrobiotic diet.

Before I begin, I would like to emphasize how much I suffered and, above all, under what conditions: (1) alone; (2) without money; and (3), even worse and terrible, to fight many obstacles at the moment as much cruel as painful. And I think to admit that it is necessary to realize the degrees of suffering of this horrible sickness. I will not speak about the moment when I suffered the most. It would be too long and cruel. I complain of terrible headaches and dripping of pus in the back of the throat and through the nose. I had to see many doctors and included specialist professors, and each one gave a different diagnosis. It was no longer a head that I had upon my shoulders but an infernal box. I have swallowed pounds of medicines. I was suffering all over: at first mental disease—hypernervousness, general state was completely bad, sometimes the pains were so horrible that I had to consult three different doctors a day, and how discouraging when I saw that each one had a different diagnosis. Some of them saw me as overweight and said that I had an imaginary illness.

Many times I had tears in my eyes and, believe me, it was the same as if they had given me a blow in my heart. This lasted several years. They did not want to believe me. Many times I wanted to commit suicide, but something stopped me. I don't know what; God only knows it. Anyhow, I never had believed in God, and I hated him because many people said that he was good. I asked myself why God could not stop all my tortures. Obviously, today I know "why."

What was my suffering? It was only after 19 surgical operations that they made a correct diagnosis: bone cancer in the frontal bone between the eyes. But why so many difficulties and operations? It is simple and at the same time very sad. Radiography is incapable of seeing this trouble because all that is in the bones is so difficult to distinguish. That is why doctors looked all around, especially in my poor nose, which has been murdered many times. It is too long to explain in detail.

I had to wait many years for an improvement. Believe me, I did not have very long to live because it began to attack my brain. One day, the frontal part began to swell and then, in spite of my sufferings, I was very happy because I thought that at this time they will believe that I was really sick. Immediately, I went to consult a very qualified doctor who recognized that it was something—but what? He did not know, although he was the best of the doctors I had consulted. This one decided on making an exploration and putting a drain in (a special kind of nail in the frontal bone). I kept it 8 days, and it was at this time that pus came out, not through the drain but on the side. At this time, I had no more sinus bone because he had removed it and replaced it with wax on one side and by a graft of skin from my stomach in the cavities of my sinus in place of the mucus membrane, in order to avoid too much mutilation. Otherwise, two big holes would have been made in my forehead. With this work, I was completely blind for 8 days. Of course, this operation should have never been performed. However, at that moment, it was no more a question of sinus. I still was suffering, and I still had infection with pus. Therefore, without giving any diagnosis, the doctor tried a new technique, the trepanation of the frontal bone, and this revealed the true nature of my disease. You see, Master Ohsawa, the price was very great in suffering, patience, and will power, even accepting to work only to pay the doctors and the druggists, and working while so sick.

I am a simple laborer, and it was very difficult for me to pay so much. At last, everything is over. Three months after the last operation there was new occurrence of pus. At this moment, I realized that there was no more hope. I was broken. It was adhesions. The trouble was growing around the place that had been operated on, and the medicine was not able to stop the infection or to diminish the pain. All this surgery had been done unnecessarily, and I was discouraged. My doctor made me understand that there was nothing more he could do. Now I was struggling for my life. I went vegetarian for one year, without great change. After that, I began macrobiotics. Now it is two years that I am on the diet, with which I am very delighted.

I am not only cured, but I have got many other advantages that are wonderful. The most extraordinary thing to happen is that I got a spiritual spirit, and I am frequently in contact with God. I am very happy. I vibrate in happiness with my interior Christ. I feel light and transported and, most of all, I have acquired faith. In fact, I considered myself the happiest man on Earth, much more than multi-millionaire friends. Today I would not change places with them.

Dear Master: I want to tell you that I never wanted to believe in God because I told myself that if there were a God, he would never had permitted me to suffer so. But today, I thank him. I understand now that it was necessary to accept these trials in order to come back to the righteous way. They helped me to learn so many things that most people do not know about. This is the most wonderful thing in the world.

I owe all that to the macrobiotic diet, and I tell you again: thank you Ohsawa!

You know me very slightly. I stayed quiet to work on myself, to judge, and then apply what was good for myself, always following your principles. Now I am free of everything, and I am very happy. Also, do not forget that I was always thinking of you, as I am today. I admire very much your courage in dealing with people who cannot accept your principles. It is sad.

I admire you because you give your life to save as many human lives as possible. I would be very pleased if you would tell all my beloved American friends that they have to open their eyes and ears and their heart so that they do not follow the same road as I, but gain health and happiness. My way was too cruel! I cannot describe how much I suffered: it was too painful. In order to avoid all this, they must have all confidence in you and apply the macrobiotic diet. Would you tell them that it is a little Frenchman that loves them with his whole heart in spite of the fact that he does not know them and that I send them my best regards. I would be happy to know that they are happier than I am.

Of the 19 operations that I had, I had two in the stomach, one in the intestines, and the rest in the head.

As you know, my dear Master, all the doctors were wrong, but I am not angry with them. They are unhappy people because they are still at the mercy of the sickness themselves. In my opinion, they are ignorant of nature. I commend them to our Eternal Father in order that they can accept the macrobiotic as soon as possible: the diet of miracles!

Personally, I thank you again a thousand times for my cure and, thanks to you, many people will be saved from death and suffering.

Please accept all my gratitude and my best thoughts of love in Christ, without forgetting Mrs. Ohsawa.

A pupil that you know very little of, but who was following you step by step.

I had a chance to listen to your interesting lectures and to read your books.

– Jacques Imbert

Letters Giving Thanks

George Ohsawa

I met George Ohsawa in the summer of 1965. The occasion was "Camp Satori," sponsored by the old Ohsawa Foundation and held in the Feather River country. Having done some reading on Zen Buddhism, I was embarrassed by the camp's name. Satori is a state achieved after many years of rigorous discipline—not after only ten days of good eating.

Mr. Ohsawa lectured three times a day. A book from the Life Science series on the structure of matter was his first text. He was jubilant that at last western scientists recognized what eastern philosophers had long ago realized: that at its most basic level, matter was nothing, and he was amused that this realization brought despair to many western minds.

I enjoyed Mr. Ohsawa's blunt English and his profound sense of humor. While apologizing for his lack of English speaking skills, he communicated very well with short phrases or often just a snort of a laugh. The latter arose when we gave him our pitiful answers to his questions. There was no hiding your ignorance at his classes; he made everyone answer.

His classes were perplexing to me. An honor roll student through high school and college, I had always been able to play the academic game quite easily. I would figure out what the teacher wanted, and give it to him. But how could I give Mr. Ohsawa "correct" answers when I couldn't begin to figure out what he wanted. I had never encountered such enigmas before. For the first time in my life I felt stupid.

My wife and I had been trying to eat macrobiotically less than a year. I had not been sick nor had I been a user of drugs except for moderate amounts of alcohol and caffeine. Previously, we had eaten an organic diet with honey in place of sugar and little blood meat. At the camp, the food was delicious and the climate hot and dry; our systems changed rapidly away from yin.

The days passed. After morning and afternoon lectures, my wife and I bathed in the clear and cold waters of the camp creek, which descended through the camp and had natural hanging gardens on the giant white granite boulders it flowed over. My wife stopped sleeping in the camper bus and joined me under the stars. We began to get glimmerings of meanings from Ohsawa's talks.

He showed us how to sit in zazen, stressing its importance. His wife demonstrated hand healing and massage. Mr. & Mrs. Ohsawa like to take pre-breakfast walks, I discovered one morning when I was walking.

The camps in those days were quite expensive compared to now, as people were hired to cook and clean up. During the camp, the grounds around the lodge got messy. I thought about picking up some of the litter, but years of habit allowed me to leave it for someone else to take care of. After all, there were paid employees there. When someone else did take care of it, he was George Ohsawa! I rounded the corner of the lodge one morning, and there was the Sensei, the Master, sweeping away and doing a good job in spite of someone following him and asking him questions. I was very moved by his doing this clean-up. I started picking up litter and trimming overgrown bushes along the trails, and at the end of the camp I mopped the lodge's main floor—to the surprise of the paid workers.

At the last lecture of the last day, Mr. Ohsawa was returning our written answers to some questions he had posed. He said he had been disillusioned with our lack of comprehension, but finally he could detect some growth. One question had been, "What is your revolutionary response to 'That which has a beginning has an end'?"

The Sensei read the answer he rated highly. He put an "X" on poor answers, one circle for adequate, two circles for good, and in one case he had drawn three concentric circles. Saying that this answer made the camp worthwhile to him, he asked whose it was. I raised my hand. "You?" he asked incredulously, remembering my earlier ignorant answers. "You are the author?" Then he asked to keep it; I made a copy before giving it to him.

When I had written my answer, I had at last managed to get beyond academic thinking. No longer seeking the rational, out of desperation, my mind expanded—I took a larger view. Here it is:

"For the first time, I see that the technological rise of the West can end in something other than disaster, whether big bang or ecological strangulation. If man began to violate the natural order, to attempt the domination of nature, he will stop doing so.

My job must be to study this beginning to seek ways of transmuting the violation. A more difficult job I cannot imagine. It is almost like a leaf floating on a great river saying, 'I shall reverse the flow'."

George Ohsawa particularly like the last sentence. As we drove down the rice-growing valley towards home, we were very grateful for the Sensei's teaching, and for the presence of his beautiful wife, Lima, who had so enjoyed seeing our baby daughter. We seemed very different people from the ones who had driven up the valley ten days before. Perhaps the camp was not so badly named after all.

– Mathew Davis

I Need You Less, Ohsawa

I met George Ohsawa at Mayaro Lodge in 1965. I can describe my experiences with him personally, from where I was at with myself then, and now, and objectively, as he stood alone as a person and human being.

When we arrived at Mayaro, I had "walking pneumonia." After a week of macrobiotic eating, cold water swims, and macrobiotic thinking, I felt so high I could touch the stones and trees, and feel the life movement in them, but I left with another cold and fever.

Until my adoption of macrobiotics, I saw illness as a siege of outside forces beyond my control. I took up macrobiotics with blind faith and a rigid application, which had severe consequences for myself and our, then new, baby. I grasped at macrobiotics as I did so many things, hoping to be "saved." But because at that time there was still no inner, deep transformation in spirit, mind, and feeling, I was not completely "cured."

Ohsawa asked deep searching questions at the Mayaro camp. "What is truth?" and "What is happiness?" All my life I had accepted what parents, teachers, friends, told me—who I was, what I was to do, think, feel. Ohsawa was asking me to think and feel for myself. He was very intrigued and amused by our attempts to answer profound questions. But I felt he alone had the only correct answer. We would chase our tails awhile. Then he would drop his answer, and it would fall like a stone into a deep pool. We would all feel the vibrations. They were good and true answers, and I tried to make them mine too. As I remember this now, I feel Ohsawa's main message was not his answer but his insistence that we dig deeper and wider for our own answer. You can have a good definition of happiness without knowing happiness. You can "head-trip-it," but if you have a good definition and live it, live happiness and truth, then you are one, a "together" human being, as Ohsawa was. He radiated warmth with an inner lightness, emptiness, laughter. When I picture him now I feel that breath—full intake, hold, hold, hold, r-e-l-e-a-s-e.

At camp, Ohsawa read my palm and face, and said "You will have great difficulty in life; better be macrobiotic." Ohsawa welcomed difficulty, but at that time I felt like running and hiding from my difficulties, and certainly not having more.

When we arrived home after camp, I had received my subbed spiritual name, Livia, meaning "Life," and although I didn't see, know, or feel it then, they go together, difficulty and life (more abundantly).

For many years, I wanted only what I thought life should be, ought to be. I was very good at suppressing all else. Now, after various kinds of "breakdowns," I am allowing it all to come, be seen, felt, transformed. For example, in totally re-experiencing (without judgment) the anger, resentment, fear-feeling of not being loved, I can begin to feel what love there is now. The flow is unblocked at the source of difficulty, the point where I closed off because the painful reality was too much. The unblocking is re-experiencing the pain but it is a most unpainful pain—joy. There is no yin without yang, no oneness without transmutation-transformation, and we have nothing to do but allow, totally feel, and observe the miracle of love-life.

Ohsawa was totally involved in the miracle, yet an amused observer. Thank you, Ohsawa, for being you: now I am becoming me. I need you less, I accept you more.

– Livia Davis

Thank You, George Ohsawa!

When I first met George Ohsawa, I saw him to be quite stern, all-knowing, salty, a man of two moods, one of seriousness, the other of humour. The things I remember and write about here picture him as I needed him to be. I often wonder how different he was, and how different I would experience him if I were to meet him today. Looking back, I realize how flexible he was and how many and varied were the facets of his personality. Every contact with him, whether in person or through correspondence, or through telepathic oneness, was a learning experience.

I remember a time that George showed what appeared to be a sternness that surpassed any I had ever heard of before. A friend of mine was working very hard, helping many other people who were trying to cure their illness. Long hours of work were very yangizing, and she was not always aware when this happened. One time she was anxiously awaiting a letter from George in answer to some questions she had written him, when lo and behold, the letter was returned unopened in an envelope neatly addressed by George, accompanied by a note that pointed out the stamp on her letter hurriedly placed upside down, and an envelope tastefully graced with marks of food. She laughed and then she cried. Once more, George with a penchant for order and balance, had taught her a new facet of macrobiotic awareness. But, oh, the delay. Having to mail back the letter and then await a returning answer!

We looked on George with awe. Many of us were having emotional and social problems. We centered everything on food—all our thoughts and conversation and activity revolved around food. I for one was scared to death of sugar and fruit, and of food in general, fearing that I would never discover the secret of balance. I hardly ever ate in a restaurant. I wanted to talk to George about the problems that were besetting me, but when I had an opportunity to approach him I always felt that he must be too busy to talk to me about the reactions I and others were having to salt, rice, and other grains in such large proportions in our diet.

One evening, after a lecture, a friend invited me to a restaurant, saying that she was dying to have a piece of apple pie and a cup of coffee. I was so turned-on by the lecture George gave that evening that I felt like going on No. 7, so I said no. The next morning she called to tell me that who should be seated at the counter eating pumpkin pie and drinking coffee, but George He asked her to join him, smiled, and asked her what she would like to have, telling her to order anything she like. Yes, you guessed, very demurely she ordered dry rye toast and a cup of tea. When her order was served she put some salt on her toast and quietly chewed and c-h-e-w-e-d her dry, salted, rye toast (while thinking about apple pie and coffee, no doubt).

The stories about George range from the wild to the ridiculous to the hilarious and the woolly. He was all of them, and then some. Most of all he was a man of humour, understanding, love, joy, and gratitude. For many of us, coming from lives that were sadly lacking in expressing appreciation and gratitude, it was difficult to fully appreciate how great the gift he gave us, and how deep should be our appreciation and gratitude. After 11 years of macrobiotics, I am just beginning to discover what it is to feel gratitude, and now I know George in a way I never could experience him before. So, I say, thank you George Ohsawa for giving me, and us, so much.

– Barbara Grace

I Gave You the Key, Now Open the Door!

There were three George Ohsawa summer camps. We had started macrobiotics seven months before the first one in Chico. Our rigid and conceptual understanding made these seven months very difficult. Everything we did was trying to follow the letter of the "law" as set down in the old edition of *Zen Macrobiotics*. Those were the days without Erewhon's sesame butter, pure and simple apple butter, or Chico-San Yinnies, etc. It was gomasio (4:1), buckwheat, and rice. Faith made us continue.

As we drove to camp, we were filled with all kinds of expectations about this Japanese man. How could any man live up to these far-out teachings? His presence fortified all our early faith. Tranquility, great depth, a humming in a wild virgin forest, something nonstop like water. His gaze penetrated to one's core. He did not ask you if you were macrobiotic; he just looked at your face, felt the tip of your nose between his thumb and index finger, shook your hand, and lingered on its fleshy areas. His most blunt comments at a consultation were punctuated with humor. He constantly talked about the "nobility" of face that is so accessible to a macrobiotic. There is no hierarchy of beauty (Hollywood), of wealth, of intellect, only hierarchy of blood, blood, blood, blood, blood.

His lectures were a stream of questions, leading you but never answering straight forward. A continuous dialogue, a hammering about everything. If someone knew why some babies have two spirals, he forbade that it be told to those who were not capable of understanding why. When I wrote to him in Tokyo to ask him what to do about our two-year-old daughter with a serious kidney infection, he wired back: "I gave you the key. Now open the door. Be smart!"

Be smart! Understand transmutation, nonstop transmutation! He called western vegetarians "protesting meat-eaters." To someone in the lecture room who coughed and showed great signs of annoyance at cigarette smoking, he wagged his finger and said, "You are arrogant—very arrogant!" "Why, Mr. Ohsawa?" "You are biologically arrogant. Your imbalance has weakened you, and now everybody has to be inconvenienced. Be independent of everything and everybody. Then you'll be free. To change the quality of your blood, regain your salt constitution of millions of years ago. Then you'll be free, and you'll make others free." His most striking saying at that time was, "One does not eat for oneself; one eats for others."

His admiration for Ueshiba was supreme. There was a man who put the unique principle to daily practice and, through love, conquered his opponent. Ohsawa always said he too was a judo man but practicing only the Do. Aikido and macrobiotics have no need for muscles to convince.

He laughed a great deal telling us the story of his tropical ulcers in Lambarene, his eating of salt wrapped in nori (in yang Africa, too!!), to cure them, and his subsequent visit to India. It was there that his disciple, seeing him consume great quantities of fruit, slavishly simulated the master and dropped dead a few days later. Ha! Ha! Ha! Ha! "How amusing."

He told us once that what most inspired his understanding was Sun Tzu's *Chinese Strategy of Love* (more commonly entitled *The Art of War*): (1) That which is supple and firm will develop constantly; (2) that which is weak and supple will be dispossessed; (3) that which is weak and powerful will become more and more celebrated and famous; and, (4) that which is strong and powerful will succumb sooner or later.

– Joe Arseguel

Ohsawa is Not Dead!

Ohsawa is not dead! As the bishop intoned the memorial chant, and we along with him, one could feel him hovering just above us in the mists of space with his rather malicious chuckle, saying, "Ha, ha, ha! He died s-o-o-o y-o-u-n-g. V-e-r-y in-terr-est-ting!" His own death must amuse him.

He is not dead, not only because we are here to follow his lead, but because a spirit as vital and intense as his can be only a living reality. He was the most electric of all men. Charismatic, an intelligence constantly at work. In his own language "smart." In palpitating 100 degrees Chico or rough Big Sur country, he was always erect, energetic, elegant. He was a presence! When you were in his company, you knew you were with the master.

Many found his method of instruction difficult. This way he had of forcing you to probe into the yin and yang of things. I did and, although at each of the three succeeding summer camps my judgment seemed to have improved, I more than once found myself trying to appear invisible. And, yet at the end of each camp there I was, miraculously revitalized. The master had given me of his own magnetism, and hopefully I was growing closer to him.

– Mimi Arseguel

Appendix

Love and Sex
Yin and Yang Game of Life

Without food, there is no life. Consequently, every phenomenon directly connected with life is the end result of food: growth, strength and weakness, bigness and smallness, wisdom and stupidity, ideology, emotional and physical activities, personal and social life, rise and fall of nations, etc.

Of course, love and marriage are no exception. They are ruled by food. According to an ancient proverb, nothing in human life exceeds the desire for food and sex. We can survive with or without sex, but without food we cease to exist. Because food is vital to us, the need for food is with us as long as we live. If you want to test how strong this desire is, try fasting for awhile.

Sexual desire comes next. It is said that all historical heroes (worldly and successful men) had strong sexual desires. For some men, sexuality is a magnetic pole that can pull them off a throne, away from an empire. Many warriors lost battles because of this strong magnetic force.

Because we desire food, our life continues. We can be thankful for this desire. How marvelous it is to have a healthy appetite! Those who enjoy meager foods possess a truly genuine appetite and are blessed with an excellent well-being. We must constantly put ourselves in this state in order to enjoy life. The aim of macrobiotic eating is to teach you to acquire this state or condition.

If you observe the macrobiotic way of eating, a genuine and natural desire for the opposite sex will spring up within you. This force may be called "sexual desire," as the ancients called it, or "love" as we call it nowadays. Without sexual desire, the human species would be exterminated, just as there would be no living existence without the desire for food. Our life begins with hunger for food. Almost instantly, from the moment of birth, babies cry for milk. Such is the desire for survival!

The desire to learn comes next, at age 7 or 8, and we become aware of the opposite sex. Menstruation starts usually at 12 to 14 for girls, and physical changes preparing for manhood come to boys around the age of 16. A healthy female becomes physically fully-equipped for motherhood at the age of 21, and a healthy male has sexual desire as a man around the age of 24. This is a natural phenomenon. Of course, there are slight variations according to different climates and races, but, ordinarily, these are the ages. Everybody has sexual desire, even those who are incapable of spiritual love. If one is without sexual desire, he is a sick man.

With the female, physical and emotional changes occur at multiples of seven, i.e., at the ages of 7, 14, 21, et seq., and with the male at multiples of eight, i.e., at 8, 16, 24. et seq. This fact is very profound and interesting from the point of view of the Unique Principle and natural medicine. This law of multiples continues for the rest of our lives. At 28, women are fully grown and are at the height of their sexual desire: they begin to stabilize at the age of 35, proceeding to a more stable emotional life at 40. Menstruation stops about the age of 49, thus ending the reproductive life of women, and their life enters into a more peaceful and deeper spiritual life.

At 32, men reach the prime of their lives. They should establish the foundation of their life work during this period. At 40, their life begins to take a calmer tone, and those who led a decadent or rough life begin to age rapidly from 40 on. A deeper spiritual life begins at 48, and at the age of 56, men enjoy the harvest of their life work. They are freed from sexual life at the age of 64, to lead a more peaceful and deeper spiritual life.

For both the male and female, six times as much as their special age circuit (seven and eight years) is the borderline of their sexual life and spiritual one. That is to say, the female at 42, and male at 48, take a high jump from a limited physical world to the life of infinite freedom.

This world is shining with peace, happiness, and freedom. Although all of us, without exception, go through the chronological age change, most people, however, do not reach this spiritual happiness. Unhappy is the man who cannot enter this Seventh Heaven of infinite freedom and who has to lead a life of greedy worldly desires. All worldly desires on this earth are based upon craving for food and sexual desire.

The Oriental custom of "boys and girls should be seated separately after the age of 7" is a mere application of the Unique Principle. Biologically speaking, girls are yang, and number seven is yang. Boys are yin and the number eight is yin. Therefore, girls start changing as early as the age of 7, and boys begin their period of change at 8. Around that time, girls start to become feminine, boys masculine. Thus, from this time, if girls and boys are reared separately, girls become more yin, and boys become more yang. If this procedure is followed, twice times seven for girls (14 years), and twice times eight for boys (16 years), both yin and yang reach their peak. So that when a girl and boy, or a man and woman, meet these two elements come closer because they have the strongest attraction toward each other. That is to say, they cannot part from each other.

This is the happiest form of marriage. Therefore, the Oriental teaching that girls and boys should never sit together after the age of 7 has a tremendous significance in terms of achieving a happy reunion in later years. This power of attraction, or force of attracting each other, is the strongest when boys are very yang and girls are very yin. (This yin does not mean physical but spiritual or metaphysical.) The more one attracts the opposite sex, the more one is at the height of his or her growth (yin and yang). Consequently, if one is not attracted by the other sex, something is wrong with him. That is to say, in the process of his growth, something was wrong with his diet.

Sex (love) is as natural a desire as the desire for food. To kill this desire is against the law of nature. It is just as hypocritical to say that love is divine as it is to say that love is evil. I repeat, love is a natural phenomenon.

Yang is centripetal and yin is centrifugal. In love, male (yang) is always an aggressive factor, and female (yin) is passive. This is the ideal way of love. When the male enters his second manhood, his yang tendency becomes more apparent, and his worldly desire, i.e., desire for business, success, and possessiveness become so powerful that he becomes a pragmatist. On the contrary, with the female, her spiritual and idealistic tendency becomes stronger and she pursues idealism. So, the way in which the male and female seek each other takes different forms.

During this period of seeking each other's company, man is like a hunter after his prey—a hunting dog whose eyes see nothing but the rabbit. The female is the pursued rabbit running into the forest (yin). The faster the hunting dog can run the better hunter he is; the faster the rabbit can run, the better off she is. A dog who does not chase a rabbit when he sees one, or the rabbit that does not run when she sees the dog, are both sick.

Furthermore, the rabbit that approaches a dog must be insane. She is either a wolf in rabbit's clothing, or is made of ice. The former might devour her husband after marriage, or kill him completely, and the latter might melt and disappear after marriage.

Only those who know these secrets can be successful in love. In the Orient, there are many sayings about love. "Love is beyond understanding." "There is no boundary for love." "If you're in love, 400 miles become four." "Love, thy name is rascal." And, "For a lover, even pock marks become dimples." As you can see, love is truly blind.

From the moment you begin to want the opposite sex, the horizon of your life becomes broader. It is the beginning of a more complex life. Since the beginning of human history, there have been numerous stories and occurrences of happy, tragic, beautiful, or ugly love. In ancient Japanese literature such as *Manyoshu, Tales of Gen-*

ji, and *Tales of Ise*, you will find torture, sufferings, tragedy, all in regard to the eternal force of love. In the later literature of Saikaku and Chikamatsu, there is found an almost suffocating kind of love. In all these books, love was painted as strong as dynamite and as fierce as lightning. But when we read them now, after hundreds of years, love appears so transitory. Love emotions are like the forms of running water in the river.

Nevertheless, love is a miracle. Without love, life is a desert, a colorless, flat, arid plain. Love, the possessive desire, gives color to life, to art it gives depth, and creates the dimensional world of pain and joy. It is most vital that we direct this love emotion onto the right path. If you misdirect or twist into detour this steering gear of love, your life will be a miserable one.

In order to attain the happy and right kind of love, correct diet is essential. The right type of love is forceful, yet natural; strong, yet gentle as a spring breeze. In order to achieve this kind of love, correct diet in youth is the first step. If you eat too many sweets, meats, and animal products, you will either become impotent or a sexual maniac in one form or another.

As I have said, the correct diet produces the man with a capacity for true love. I have proven this point in my books. However, if you want other proof, read the many poems, novels, plays, histories, and autobiographies, both of the East and the West, and study the dietary history contained in them. Faithful authors usually describe or tell their heroes' and heroines' dietary taste or habits. You will learn from these histories, fictional and factual, the indivisible, inseparable connection between diet and love.

Faith—The Power of Positive Thinking
— Norman Vincent Peale

This book has a record: the best seller for 168 weeks. I have read its two millionth copy. It's wonderful. And as there are 124 million registered diseased people in this country, one must sell five to ten times more copies so that all these sick people may learn this anti-materialistic method and apply it on themselves.

The author insists upon the importance of having strong faith in God. This is not an undesirable method in this materialistic age. I don't deny its efficacy for those who can have faith. But it is impossible for those who cannot have it. And how many people have genuine faith? Here is a faint light for those who have been obliged to have faith in God after having tried modern medications at great expense for many years without any amelioration at all, and who at last were given up by medicine and condemned as physical or mental incurables. They are already mutilated chemically, and it is often too late for them. If they had been educated to have faith from the beginning, some would have avoided the endless labyrinth of drugs and surgery that is guaranteed by official medicine as the way to health. (By faith it is meant not a superstitious belief but a reverent comprehension of the Order of the Universe and obedience to these laws of life in eating and drinking; in ancient language, "prayer and fasting.") But they were all educated to have faith in education, science, government, and medicine from the very beginning.

Furthermore, the church has lost its faith in God. The church has conceded its ancient peace-health-giving function long since to the newcomer named science, and to medicine. There are so many outstanding religious people who have faith in scientific medicine-men instead of seeking cures by the hand of God. Many churches have established hospitals without any shame or humiliation. Many others are collecting money to fight against cancer. Isn't this a far cry from

Jesus' teaching? "Do not resist, even against evils!" Is Christianity no longer the teaching of Jesus? (I know there is a small church that is teaching natural cure very bravely. I hope it will grow bigger and stronger. But no one knows the true medicine of Jesus!)

I am not arguing against positive thinking that can cure sickness. I only regret that the author of this book, like so many other spiritualists and Christian Science teachers, emphasizes the importance of faith without explaining the real nature of faith that allows you to say to the mountain, "Enter into the sea." He is teaching only to "Believe" phonographically. That is to say, he is preaching only the verbal formula, not the practical truth of Jesus' medicine that can guarantee not only bodily health in this relative world but infinite freedom, eternal happiness, and absolute justice. Theory without practice is useless, practice without theory is dangerous!

Many of his readers may be cured for a time by imitating the author mechanically. But having no firm theoretical foundation of faith, they will suffer again the same disease or suffer new ones after awhile. Or else they will easily forget faith's superiority as they are simple imitation-Christians. They have been converted with a very low, egoistic, and materialistic purpose: to cure themselves for their happiness and nothing more. They have bought the Bible as they have bought drugs—through high-powered advertising.

Jesus cured many diseased people, but he never intended to establish a hospital. He could cure any disease by teaching true faith and the way to have it. And is there any Christian nowadays who can cure any disease without medication, once and forever, and not only disease but liberation from all kinds of difficulties and unhappiness forever?—and even from wars?

Mr. Peale, you have helped so many millions of people, which is really wonderful. But allow me to give you one task: Cure only one patient, "Christianity," which is being mutilated and crippled by the so-called scientific medicine!

Occidental medicine is complicating things. First of all, it has cut man in two: body and mind. And blood, too: white and red globules and so on indefinitely. The more modern medicine is developed, the more we need expensive hospitals and large pharmaceutical industries, and the more diseased people! The specialists are all desperate with their highly developed techniques, wonderful medicines, and awaiting the "God only knows medicine" according to *Time* magazine of March 7 and *Realités* of February 1960.

I have come to Europe and America as a simple old interpreter of the medicine of Jesus and his philosophy. If the author of "Positive Thinking" would kindly accept my proposition, I would do my best to give him all my secrets.

I would like to sell only 2,000 copies of my *Philosophy of Oriental Medicine* instead of two million, so that I might meet a handful of people who could understand what faith is and how one can have faith that knows nothing is impossible in this world.

Hunza Land

Land of longevity with no fatigue, no disease, no police force, and no crime! This wonderland has been known since Sir MacCarrison published his famous book *Nutrition and Health* some 40 years ago. A doctor from Nebraska visited this wonderland recently and published *Hunza Land* after his return. Unfortunately, he is not a very good observer or thinker. He failed to describe quantitatively the nutrition of these people, although he attributed all their physical and mental superiority over sick Western man to their traditional eating and way of life.

In particular, he omitted any reference to salt and its use per person per day. Chemically, a dose of salt can change blood pressure and composition, as well as kidney function, immediately, and consequently effect the entire state of health. Salt is in fact the most precious thing in Hunza Land. This omission is the basic fault of this book and its author, Dr. Banik. He failed to stress the crucial fact that sugar is unknown in this country. He could not understand deeply how important a fact this is.

The final chapter, however, "The Inspiration of Hunza," is full of good and sound thinking that will encourage many people. I hope that the author will study our macrobiotic medicine-philosophy, which is also thousands of years old.

Chewing

Chewing is most important in macrobiotics. You have no teeth in your stomach nor in the intestines. So you must chew in your mouth, 50 times per mouthful, at least. You are well-accustomed to chewing by your chewing of gum for so many years. If you have no time to chew, or if you are so busy in your business that you cannot taste quietly your food and drink, you have no qualification to step into this Macrobiotic diet.

In reality, good chewing of well-balanced food is the greatest ceremony of creating Life. You are what you are eating and drinking. This is a biological and physiological fact. If you can judge what to eat and how, according to our philosophy, you can control your health, and you will have infinite freedom, eternal happiness, and absolute justice. In this country, one considers eating and drinking as pleasure. That is the biggest and worst thing. Food must first of all be normal and righteous, according to biological and physiological laws, or difficulties will follow sooner or later. Pleasure is very important in our life. I don't deny it. But I recommend to you, after having met thousands and thousands of unhappy men, to take the best food and drink according to our thousands-of-years-old philosophy, experimented with by thousands of millions of people. You will find these so delicious that you will never give them away.

Chew every spoonful 50 times or more. The more you chew, the quicker you will master our philosophy of longevity and rejuvenation.

The True Guru Is Not Sick

In the Far East, we look up to two kinds of leaders. First, the *sensei* (meaning literally born before) includes all elders. This respect for age is the basis of our traditional Oriental society—it is natural and unforced.

Then there are the gurus, the *si, sri,* or real *sensei*, who are spiritual guides, men free from suffering and fear. The true guru is not sick physically, psychologically, or spiritually; he is Macrobiotic. He points out the way to infinite freedom, eternal happiness, and absolute integrity. Rejuvenation and longevity alone do not make the guru—he must spend his life opening the door for others. [Lao-tse says: "The strong man submits to the weaker."]

By his very nature, his vibrations, his unspoken essence, the guru convinces everyone of the way to eternal happiness (collective peace and well-being) and infinite freedom (individual freedom). His minute-to-minute life makes him loved by everybody everywhere.

In the traditional Oriental societies, a guru arrives at such a state without resorting to medicinal remedies, instruments, or weapons. He is Zen in the sense of being a cup overflowing with emptiness, without excess, not unlike the pot-bellied monk. His healing power is *wu-wei*, the unconscious by-product of his intuition. Do-goodism simply creates a welfare state of cripples, beggars, and slaves.

Are present-day Western doctors and therapists real gurus? Do they follow Jesus' example—prayer and fasting—not pills and hospitals? Even his followers sent abroad to heal had no training in symptomatic treatments. How removed from today's doctors, nurses, and other missionaries!

Christianity stripped of Jesus' medicine is no Christianity at all. Here is the origin of Western medicine's impasse. If only Christians would re-discover his Way!

Vitamins Listed from Yin to Yang

The figures are determined by the ratio of:

$$\frac{\text{Yin}}{\text{Yang}} = \frac{\text{0, N, S} \ (\text{Oxygen, Nitrogen, Sulfur})}{\text{C, H} \quad (\text{Carbon, Hydrogen})}$$

and obviously vary according to the specific source of the vitamin.

Rutin (most yin). 0.43080
C 0.42850
B_2 . . . . 0.28000
B_{12} 0.26300
Niacin 0.25000
B_1 . . . . 0.23300
B_6 . . . . 0.21500

K_3 . . . . 0.11100
A 0.03700
E 0.03570
D_3 (most yang) 0.01408

Yin and yang are like the "x" and the "y"; with them we plot points.

Basic Chemical Composition of the Human Body

(Hackh)

	%		%
O	62.43	Na	0.08000
C	21.15	Mg	0.02400
H	9.88	I	0.01400
N	3.10	F	0.00900
Ca	1.90	Fe	0.00500
P	0.95	Br	0.00200
K	0.23	Al	0.00100
S	0.16	Si	0.00100
Cl	0.08	Mn	0.00005

(Gamble)

	Sodium (mg/ml)	Potassium (mg/ml)
Plasma	350	91
Perspiration	134	39
Saliva	76	76
Gastric juices	136	36
Pancreatic juices	324	18
Intestinal juices	240	90
Feces	81	282
Urination (average food intake)	207	195
Average elimination through urine in 24 hours	3.11 gm	2.94 gm

Minerals and Yin/Yang Balance of Foods

It has often been suggested that the ratio of potassium (K) to sodium (Na) is an indication of whether a particular food is more yin or more yang, potassium being the representative yin element and sodium the representative yang element. While this ratio may often be useful as an indication, it can also be misleading as sometimes a very yin food has a lower K/Na ratio than one that is more yang.

There are six minerals that occur in most foods in larger than trace amounts. Beside the two previously mentioned, these are: magnesium (Mg), calcium (Ca), phosphorus (P) and sulfur (S). These elements can also be classified by yin and yang with the resulting grouping: Na and Mg are yang. K, Ca, P, and S are yin. We may be able to more completely express yin/yang in terms of mineral balance by determining the ratio between these elements.

$$\frac{Na+Mg}{K+Ca+P+S} \quad \frac{(Yang)}{(Yin)}$$

Almond	$\dfrac{4+270}{773+234+504+96}$	Cabbage	$\dfrac{20+13}{233+49+29+958}$
Apple	$\dfrac{1+8}{110+7+10+201}$	Carrot	$\dfrac{47+23}{341+37+36+445}$
Asparagus	$\dfrac{2+20}{278+22+62+536}$	Cherry	$\dfrac{2+14}{191+22+19+176}$
Barley	$\dfrac{3+124}{296+34+290+240}$	Chestnut	$\dfrac{641}{454+27+88+300}$
Beans, white	$\dfrac{19+170}{1196+144+425+130}$	Lentils	$\dfrac{30+80}{790+79+377+120}$
Beets	$\dfrac{60+25}{335+16+33+50}$	Rice, brown	$\dfrac{9+88}{214+32+221+10}$

[Sources for information: *Composition of Foods, USDA Handbook No. 8*, 1963, for all values except that of sulfur. *Composition and Facts About Foods*, Ford Heritage, 1968.] Values are expressed in milligrams per 100 grams edible portion. All listings are for raw foods.

Dentie: A Natural Product
(See recipe #80.)

1. For use on sore gums. After brushing teeth, rub a very small amount into the gums—and let it be absorbed.

2. For a child's toothache, put a bit inside the cavity.

3. For sore throat, cough, or adenoid flare-ups, prepare as a gargling solution.

4. For any sudden or acute inflammation or infection.

5. For other general swelling or cracking of the skin.

Used sparingly but regularly on the gums and as a gargle, dentie will prevent any local mouth and throat problems. A small envelope of dentie should last several months. All other toothpastes and powders contain chemical products, yin in nature and expensive because of their commercial origin.

Foods Listed from Yin to Yang
(A General Guide)

Fruit
dates
avocado
banana
pineapple
grape
prunes
orange
tangerine
cantaloupe
peach
pear
lemon
apricot
blueberry
blackberry
watermelon
strawberry
cherry
apple

Oil
soy oil
mayonnaise
safflower oil
olive oil
corn oil
corn germ oil

white sesame oil
black sesame oil

Alcohol
wine
vodka
whiskey
sake
beer

Nuts
cashew
peanut
pistachio
pecan
almond
walnut
chestnut

Seaweeds
nori
dulse
kelp
hiziki
wakame
kombu

Beans
soybeans
green peas
white beans
split peas
kidney beans
pinto beans
lentils
chickpeas
black beans
aduki beans

Vegetables
shiitake mushrooms
eggplant
tomato
bamboo shoot
potato
sweet potato
water chestnut
cucumber
spinach
asparagus
swiss chard
string beans
beets
cauliflower
broccoli

Chinese cabbage
celery
cabbage
lettuce
escarole
kale
daikon
radish
turnip
parsnip
scallions
leeks
pumpkin
onion
parsley
squash
garlic
watercress
coltsfoot
carrot
lotus root
burdock
jinenjo (wild)

Beverages
all sugar drinks
fruit juices
coffee
tea [dyed]
mint
camomile
bancha
kokkoh

mugwort
yannoh
mu tea
ginseng

Dairy Foods
yogurt
ice cream
butter
blue cheese
milk
camembert
gruyere
roquefort
goat milk
goat cheese

Seeds
sunflower
pumpkin
squash
sesame

Condiments
gomasio
miso
tamari
tekka
salt

Grains
corn
barley

oats
rye
whole wheat
rice
millet
buckwheat

**Fish and Animal
Foods**
oyster
clam
octopus
eel
carp
mussel
halibut
lobster
trout
sole
crab
shrimp
herring
tuna
salmon
sardine
red snapper
caviar
chicken
meat (red)
fowl
egg

Books by George Ohsawa

Acupuncture and the Philosophy of the Far East
Atomic Age and the Philosophy of the Far East
Book of Judo (The Art of Peace)
Cancer and the Philosophy of the Far East (Macrobiotics:
    The Way of Healing)
Essential Ohsawa
Four Hours to Basic Japanese
Gandhi: The Eternal Youth
Jack and Mitie
Macrobiotic Guidebook for Living
Macrobiotics: An Invitation to Health and Happiness
Order of the Universe
Philosophy of Oriental Medicine (The Book of Judgment)
Unique Principle
You Are All Sanpaku
Zen Macrobiotics

A list of books by George Ohsawa and others on macrobiotics can be obtained from the George Ohsawa Macrobiotic Foundation, PO Box 3998, Chico, CA 95927-3998; 530-566-9765; fax 530-566-9768; *gomf@earthlink.net.* Or, visit *www.ohsawamacrobiotics.com.*

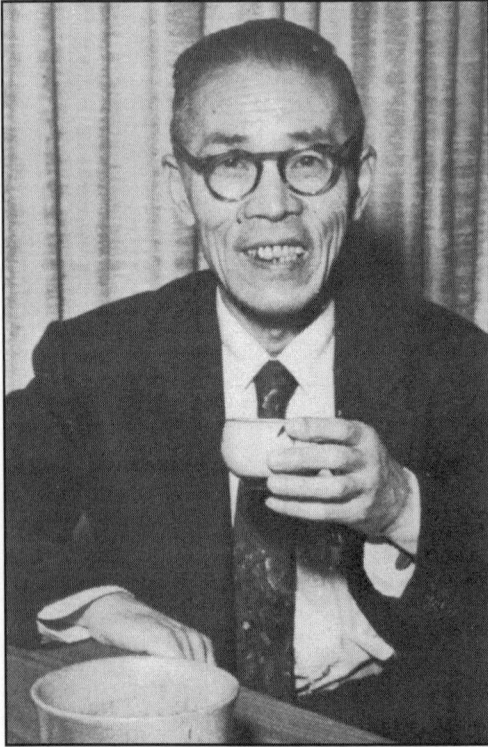

GEORGE OHSAWA

The Author

George Ohsawa (Yukikazu Sakurazawa) was born in Kyoto, the old capitol of Japan, on October 18, 1893.

He is the author of more than three hundred books, ten of which have been published in France since 1926. His work *A New Theory of Nutrition and Its Therapeutic Effect*, written and published in Japan in 1920, is in its seven-hundredth edition.

Thirty years of his life were spent introducing Oriental culture to Europe, while simultaneously interpreting the culture of the West for Japan. Among his many translations into Japanese are *Man, the Unknown* by Alexis Carrel and *The Meeting of East and West* by F. S. C. Northrup.

His passing on April 24, 1966 deeply saddened the countless individuals who are eternally indebted to him for having given to them the gift of life itself. Their infinite gratitude is expressed in a continuation of the vital work he undertook and so ably pursued for more than fifty-four years.

A list of books by George Ohsawa and others on macrobiotics can be obtained from the George Ohsawa Macrobiotic Foundation, PO Box 3998, Chico, CA 95927-3998; 530-566-9765; fax 530-566-9768; *gomf@earthlink.net*. Or, visit *www.gomf.macrobiotic.net*.

Printed in Great Britain
by Amazon.co.uk, Ltd.,
Marston Gate.